Campylobacter II

Proceedings of the Second International Workshop on Campylobacter Infections Brussels, 6 - 9 September 1983

Edited by

A. D. Pearson

Public Health Laboratory, Southampton, UK

M. B. Skirrow

Department of Microbiology (Pathology), Royal Infirmary, Worcester, UK

B. Rowe

Central Public Health Laboratory, London, UK

J. R. Davies

Public Health Laboratory Service Headquarters, London, UK

and

D. M. Jones

Public Health Laboratory, Manchester, UK

London 1983

Public Health Laboratory Service

PHLS

Published by the Public Health Laboratory Service,
61 Colindale Avenue, London NW9 5EQ

First published 1983

ISBN 0 901 14413 4

The three back cover photographs show, from the top left, "Jimmi-Juni", an untouched electron micrograph of **Campylobacter jejuni** in rabbit ileum (reproduced by courtesy of Dr Tom Frederick, Rochester Institute of Technology and Naval Medical Research Institute, Bethesda, Maryland, USA); an electron micrograph of **Campylobacter jejuni** plasmid pMAK 175 which encodes resistance to tetracycline - the plasmid size is 44.7 kb (29 x 10^6 daltons) determined with respect to pBR 322 plasmid shown at upper left (reproduced by courtesy of Dr Diane Taylor, Department of Microbiology, University of Alberta, Edmonton, Alberta, Canada); and a dividing campylobacter-like organism isolated from the gastric antrum of a patient with a duodenal ulcer (reproduced by courtesy of Dr Barry Marshall, Department of Gastroenterology, Royal Perth Hospital, Perth, Western Australia).

Printed in England by the Devon Print Group, Exeter

Contents

SESSION IV: SEROTYPING AND PHAGE TYPING: APPLICATION AND INTERPRETATION

SESSION V: PATHOGENESIS

SESSION VI: EPIDEMIOLOGY AND SURVIVAL EXPERIMENTS

Preface

The editors wish to thank the sponsors, the Scientific Organising Committee, the chairmen and rapporteurs and the presenters for their contributions to this publication.

The sponsors were the Free University of Brussels, the International Centre for Diarrhoeal Research - Bangladesh, the World Health Organisation and the Public Health Laboratory Service. The members of the Scientific Organising Committee were Dr Blaser (Denver, USA), Professor Butzler (Brussels, Belgium), Dr Feldman (Atlanta, USA), Dr Fleming (Toronto, Canada), Dr Greenough (Atlanta, USA), Dr Pearson (Southampton, UK) and Dr Skirrow (Worcester, UK). This group was assisted by Dr Lauwers (Brussels, Belgium), Dr Karmali (Toronto, Canada), Dr Rowe (London, UK), Dr Kosunen (Helsinki, Finland), Dr Taylor (Glasgow, UK) and Dr Aziz (Dhaka, Bangladesh) in chairing the discussions and providing reviews of each of the six sessions.

We would also like to thank Mrs Pat Allgood, Mrs Sarah Sparrow and Miss Elizabeth Hutcheson for their secretarial assistance.

October 1983 A. D. Pearson

List of Papers Presented

CLINICAL AND THERAPEUTIC ASPECTS

TAXONOMY, BIOTYPING, ISOLATION AND DETECTION

ANTIGENS AND SERODIAGNOSIS

SEROTYPING AND PHAGE TYPING: APPLICATION AND INTERPRETATION

PATHOGENESIS

EPIDEMIOLOGY AND SURVIVAL EXPERIMENTS

Introduction

This volume reports on and summarises the 152 oral and poster presentations given by an international group of participants at the Brussels workshop in September 1983. The volume is divided into six major sessions which reflect the sessions into which the actual workshop contributions were originally grouped. Summaries of the current state of knowledge, achievements since the First International Workshop (held at Reading, UK, in 1981) and future objectives are given by the editors and by Dr D J Taylor at the opening of each session. These reports are then followed by abstracts of every paper presented in each session. Authors were specifically requested to provide updated abstracts of their presentations at the workshop. The abstracts therefore reflect the actual and most recent information available at the time of the workshop. Finally, the volume is supplemented by a report on a special session on poultry infection which was arranged during the course of the workshop and by a bibliography of significant publications on campylobacters which have been published in the past two years or which were known to be in press at the end of September 1983.

This volume contains reports indicating that isolation and serological techniques are used widely, and that the investigation of outbreaks suggests common sources of infection which point to easily recognisable targets for preventive measures. The combination of biotyping with serotyping is a major advance in source tracing, although further work is required to provide a unified system of reporting antigenic determinants. The reports of a campylobacter-like agent from the antrum of patients with gastritis or gastric ulceration and of campylobacter-like organisms (CLOs) from homosexuals with diarrhoea will stimulate investigation of the relevance of campylobacter isolates other than **Campylobacter jejuni/coli** to human disease.

Future objectives should include the development of enrichment techniques and of chemically defined media, as well as the application of new technology to the production of DNA probes. There is clearly a need to identify and compare a limited number of carefully defined strains for use in experimental work which could assist in the identification of virulence markers. No mechanism for pathogenicity has yet been proven. This goal might best be approached by the detailed application of relevant new technologies to a carefully defined bank of isolates.

A. D. Pearson

Public Health Laboratory,
Southampton, UK

Session I

CLINICAL AND THERAPEUTIC ASPECTS

Report on the Session

CLINICAL ASPECTS

Infections due to campylobacters other than *C. jejuni* and *C. coli*

It is fitting to start this commentary by highlighting some notable developments on infection with new types of campylobacter and campylobacter-like organisms.

Much interest was shown in the report by Marshall and Warren (p. 11), from Western Australia, of the colonisation of the stomach antrum of patients with peptic ulceration and gastritis by spiral bacteria. These bacteria were first noticed by Dr Warren in histological sections of gastric antrum [1]. They were not obvious in sections stained with haematoxylin and eosin, but showed up clearly with Warthin-Starry silver staining. Their association with pathological lesions is impressive. They were found in 100% of patients with duodenal ulcer, 80% of patients with gastric ulcer and 95% of patients with "active chronic gastritis". By contrast they were found in only two of 31 control patients. Enormous numbers of bacteria were seen in association with the lesions. They were present between the cells of the surface epithelium and there was superficial infiltration with polymorphonuclear neutrophil leucocytes. The bacteria were absent or rare where there were no signs of gastric or duodenal inflammation.

How do these bacteria withstand gastric acidity? The answer is simple: they colonize the mucosal surface beneath the layer of mucus that is normally present and across which there is a steep pH gradient. This emphasises the difference that can exist between surface mucosal and general luminal flora, a difference long appreciated by veterinary microbiologists, but less so by medical microbiologists mainly because it is difficult to obtain mucosal samples from human patients. However, endoscopy is now permitting new approaches to be made. Lee **et al.** (p. 112) put forward the hypothesis that spiral bacteria are specially adapted to viscous environments owing to their characteristic form of motility, and that **C. jejuni** is a surface-associated organism – at least in the mouse intestine.

Marshall and Warren described two clinical features of particular interest. First, biopsy of patients who had relapsed after treatment with cimetidine showed an increased intensity and extent of colonisation (to the whole stomach). Second, treatment with bismuth in the form of De-Nol® (tripotassium dicitrato bismuthate) caused a disappearance of the bacteria and of local inflammation, though they reappeared after cessation of treatment. Like most other oxidase-positive bacteria (including campylobacters), these organisms are very sensitive to bismuth in vitro. Antacids had no effect on colonisation.

These bacteria can be seen in Gram-stained smears and cultured from biopsy material or brushings of the gastric antrum of infected patients. Moist plain chocolate or blood agar as well as campylobacter selective agar should be inoculated and incubated under microaerobic conditions for at least 3 days at 37 °C (these bacteria do not grow at 25 or 42 °C). Just before this workshop a positive culture was obtained at the Worcester Royal Infirmary, UK, from a woman with gastric ulcer and hiatus hernia. She was the first patient sampled by Dr Marshall who was attending a gastroscopy clinic as a guest of Dr N. H. Dyer; so the bacteria are not exclusively Australian.

The taxonomic status of these organisms is discussed on p. 36. The burning question is whether they are of primary or secondary importance in the aetiology of peptic ulceration. That high priority should be given to finding an answer goes without saying. A study of immune response and the results of treatment directed against the organisms would be useful approaches.

Other new campylobacter-like organisms (CLOs) were reported in association with proctitis in homosexual men in Seattle, USA. In fact three groups of CLOs (described by Fennell **et al.**, p. 47) are implicated. Again there is an association with disease in that they were isolated from 28 of 181 symptomatic homosexual men compared with seven of 77 asymptomatic homosexual men and none of 150 normal heterosexual men and women, but their role is not clear. The presenters claimed to have shown a serological response to the bacteria in men with proctitis, and a strain of CLO-1 was isolated from the blood of one patient. That these CLOs have been overlooked until now might be explained by the fact that all isolations were made from specimens taken by proctoscopy; they have not been cultured from faeces. This is yet another example of the necessity to consider mucosal as opposed to luminal flora in the pathogenesis of disease. The origin of these bacteria is completely unknown. It is intriguing to speculate whether the appearance of these bacteria in such a specific group of people might signify a breakdown of immunity heralding the onset of acquired immune deficiency syndrome (AIDS).

Turning to a more familiar organism, Heinzer (p. 12) suggested that **C. fetus** subsp. **fetus** might be a more important cause of febrile enteritis than had been thought. (It is usually associated with systemic infection in compromised patients rather than acute enteritis.) He pointed out that not all campylobacter selective media are appropriate for the isolation of **C. fetus** (as opposed to **C. jejuni**) even if cultures were incubated at 37 °C instead of 42 °C. Skirrow's medium gave the best results but Campy-BAP was unsuitable. Although Dr Heinzer reported the isolation of **C. fetus** from 12 patients (**C. jejuni** from 214 patients in the same period), Professor Butzler quoted Dr Kasper of Mannheim as having cultured 23,000 specimens of faeces without a single isolation of **C. fetus**. The general feeling was that extra cultures incubated at 37 °C were not worthwhile. In answer to a question about **C. fetus** subsp. **venerealis**, Dr Fleming said that this organism had been isolated from the blood of a child with a mild febrile illness in the Hospital for Sick Children, Toronto. As far as we know this is the first proven instance of this subspecies causing infection in a human being.

Infections due to **C. jejuni** and **C. coli**

The human volunteer experiments reported by Black and his colleagues (p. 13) were of outstanding interest. Two strains of **C. jejuni**, both isolated from outbreaks of campylobacter enteritis, were given to volunteers in graded doses and the number and volume of stools recorded. Several interesting results came out of this study, among which were the following:

(1) Symptomatic infection could result from a dose of 400-800 bacteria, but symptomless infection or no infection could follow the ingestion of much larger numbers.

(2) More patients became infected when the bacteria were given in a solution of sodium bicarbonate than in milk.

(3) The incubation period to fever was 68 h and to diarrhoea 88 h.

(4) The two strains of **C. jejuni** produced illness of different

severity.

(5) When suspensions of bacteria from spreading and non-spreading (subsequently shown to be non-flagellate) colonies of a single strains were given together, only spreading colonies were seen on culture of faeces.

(6) No isolation was made from blood despite frequent sampling.

(7) Volunteers were resistant to reinfection with the same strain.

Experiments of this type are clearly capable of providing valuable information that cannot be obtained in any other way. During the ensuing discussion, Dr Lee (New South Wales, Australia) and Dr Blaser (Denver, USA) criticised the popular concept of an infective dose as being of a finite size. There were too many variables, such as the nature and volume of stomach contents and nature of inoculum, to allow such a concept. The most one could say was that the larger the dose the greater the number of people who were likely to become ill. Dr Lee pointed out that this was of more than theoretical interest because a simple statement that an organism has a low infective dose can be misunderstood and lead to inappropriate action being taken by health officials.

An interesting account of the impact of an outbreak of campylobacter enteritis affecting 189 of 785 boys at a boarding school was given by Hoskins and Davies (p. 14). This was a sharp outbreak of short duration attributed to the consumption of accidentally unpasteurized milk (epidemiology described by Wilson **et al.**, p. 143). Over 90% of boys had fever, but not for more than 48 h. Abdominal pain commonly preceded diarrhoea and several boys had fever and abdominal pain without diarrhoea. Vomiting was reported by less than 10% of the boys and only one had blood in his stools. Boys who became ill first, i.e. those who had the shortest incubation period, had a higher incidence of fever and more severe illness than those reporting sick later in the outbreak. Some boys had abdominal tenderness, but none had it to a degree that suggested acute appendicitis. An unusually large number of boys (12) had urticaria, but it was not known what relationship, if any, this had to campylobacter infection. Of particular interest is that of 12 boys who were affected in a similar outbreak of campylobacter enteritis two years previously, in 1980, 10 were also infected in the current outbreak. This indicates that any immunity gained in the first outbreak was either shortlived or else there was no cross-immunity between the two infecting strains (which were of different serotypes).

A study of travellers' diarrhoea affecting visitors to Bangladesh (Speelman **et al.**, see p. 14) leaves no doubt that many endemic strains of **C. jejuni** are pathogenic to people normally resident in Europe and North America. The clinical picture was often similar to shigellosis. In Bangladesh, symptomless infection, notably in children, is very common and it had been suggested that many strains were non-pathogenic or of low virulence.

Several presentations concerned infection in children, especially children in developing countries. In contrast to the Bangladesh findings, De Mol and Habyaremye (p. 16) reported a clear association between the isolation of **C. jejuni** and diarrhoea in Rwanda, at least in children less than 1 year old (25% of all infections). This association became less clear with advancing age, until over the age of 3 years there was no difference in isolation rate between children with and without diarrhoea. The clinical features of children with **C. jejuni** diarrhoea were not significantly different from those with diarrhoea not associated with **C. jejuni**, except for a higher body temperature in the **C. jejuni** group. There were two epidemiological points of note. First, most campylobacter infections were encountered in the dry season and beginning of the rainy season. Second, there were more **C. jejuni**-infected domestic animals in families containing a **C. jejuni**-infected person than in families not containing an infected person (the total number of animals in the two groups was essentially the same).

In a report from South Africa (Soweto) by Richardson **et al.** (p. 15), **C. jejuni** was found most often in children between 1 and 3 years of age, but there was a significant association with diarrrhoea only in children below the age of 1 year. The incidence of infection did not seem to be affected by either breast or supplemented feeding, or by nutritional state. Diarrhoea tended to be watery; blood was rarely present. Many children had a low grade fever. Family studies detected spread of infection only when the index case had been a child of less than 3 years of age. Isolation of several serotypes of **C. jejuni** from single patients over a period of several weeks or months indicated that sequential or mixed infections were common. Excretion of the same serotype for up to 13 weeks was also observed, but whether such instances represent unduly prolonged excretion (relative to that in technically advance countries) is not clear. If there is genuine prolongation of excretion in Sowetan children, then an explanation is required. Children with severe campylobacter diarrhoea did not excrete for longer than average. Prolonged excretion, however, was certainly a feature of **C. jejuni** infection in immunodeficient children studied by Melamed **et al.** in Israel (p. 21).

The possibility of simultaneous infection with more than one serotype was studied by Lauwers and De Vuyst (p. 17). They followed the pattern of excretion in children for up to 17 months. Isolations obtained from a patient more than 1 month apart were usually of different serotypes and probably indicated sequential infection. On the other hand, 12.8% of patients sampled repeatedly within 14 days harboured strains of more than one serotype, and they probably had true mixed infections even though all attempts to detect multiple serotypes among the colonies of a single culture were unsuccessful.

Hanslo **et al.** (p. 16), also from South Africa (Cape Town), reported an extraordinarily large number (63) of children with bacteraemia detected over 5 years. Three-quarters of them were less than 1 year old and half of them were judged to be malnourished. Most isolations were obtained only on terminal subculture of the Castaneda type medium (50 ml) after 10 days incubation. All isolates were **C. jejuni** or **C. coli**, none were **C. fetus.** Strains were of no particular serotype, but the proportion of **C. coli** was slightly higher than was found normally in stools. Chemotherapy appeared to have little effect on the course of illness. How does one explain this high incidence of bacteraemia, which is all the more remarkable in view of the limited amounts of blood obtainable from infants? It is unlikely that it is purely a matter of technique, though this is probably one factor. Perhaps the figures are high simply because a large number of cultures were taken (we were not told how many). Malnourishment in early infancy may be an important factor.

The results of a prospective study designed to assess the role of gastrointestinal pathogens in children with appendicitis or suspected appendicitis was the subject of a presentation by Pearson **et al.** (p. 19). Serological evidence of campylobacter infection occurring at the time of hospital admission was found in no less than 8.5% of children with proven appendicitis and a further 3% had evidence of recent infection. These figures were based on the detection of rising and falling titres of IgG antibody to **C. jejuni/coli** by ELISA, and the authors were careful to point out that further work is required to assess the significance of these results by the use of a parallel and preferably more specific test. Nevertheless, the possibility that **C. jejuni** and **C. coli** could be a cause of even a minority of acute appendicitis cases is an important one. It is interesting that fewer children suffering from abdominal pain without appendicitis - a syndrome known to be associated with campylobacter infection - had serological evidence of infection (6%) than those with appendicitis.

The post-mortem findings in six fatal cases of campylobacter infection in children in Bangladesh were presented by Butler **et al.** (p. 19). In some cases inflammatory and ulcerative lesions in the small and large bowel probably contributed to death, but other pathogens were thought to have played a dominant role.

Velasco **et al.** (p. 21) described relatively mild illness with absence of fever in neonates infected with **C. jejuni**. This is something that has been described previously. All infected infants recovered without specific treatment. The authors stated that jaundice was more frequently observed in infected than uninfected infants. They also stated that they had clear evidence (not presented) that some infections in a creche were due to cross-infection from nurses.

There were no presentations on gestational infections in women, but this is an appropriate point to draw attention to a report by Kist **et al.** [2] of a case of **C. coli** septicaemia associated with septic abortion. It is interesting on two counts: it is the first recognised instance of **C. coli** (as opposed to **C. jejuni** or **C. fetus**) being implicated in septic abortion and it summarises the published reports of campylobacter-associated abortions that have appeared to date (more in the last three years than in all years to 1980).

THERAPEUTIC ASPECTS

Antimicrobial sensitivities and sensitivity testing

Several studies of in vitro sensitivities of **C. jejuni** and **C. coli** were presented. Michel and Rogol (p. 24) reported almost 15% of strains resistant to erythromycin and 41% resistant to tetracycline in Israel. These resistant strains belonged to several serotypes, but 70% of strains resistant to erythromycin were on one serotype. Resistance to both drugs was distributed about equally between **C. jejuni** and **C. coli**, in contrast to the pattern in Europe and North America, where erythromycin resistance is almost confined to **C. coli**.

Sensitivity to erythromycin, clindamycin and various other antimicrobial agents was the subject of a presentation by Wang **et al.** (p. 24). They reported differences in sensitivity between strains of **C. coli** isolated from human patients and pigs. They also detected differences in sensitivity to clindamycin, erythromycin, rosaramicin and Sch 32063 between **C. coli** and **C. jejuni**. Further differences in sensitivity between these two species were described by Smith **et al.** (p. 29). Most of their (Canadian) strains of **C. coli** were highly resistant to streptomycin, whereas all 22 strains of **C. jejuni** were sensitive (MIC $\leq$ 4 mg/l).

Felmingham **et al.** (p. 25) showed that six newly synthesized quinoline derivatives were more active than nalidixic acid against **C. jejuni**. The most active compounds, ciprofloxacin and DL 8280, had MIC_{90} values of 0.25 mg/l compared with 8.0 mg/l for nalidixic acid. These compounds are bactericidal and can be taken orally; blood concentrations of 2–5 mg/l can probably be attained. They may well find a place in the therapy of campylobacter enteritis, but it must be emphasised that they are contraindicated in children since they affect growing cartilage.

Rodriguez-Gonzalez **et al.** (p. 26) reported that cefotaxime and ceftriaxone were the least inactive of seven cephalosporins against **C. jejuni**. The cephalosporins are not antibiotics that would normally be used for the treatment of **C. jejuni** infections, though they might be considered for infections with **C. fetus**, which is a more sensitive organism.

Clinical trials

Mandal and Ellis's paper (p. 27) was the only one to report a clinical therapeutic trial – a double-blind trial of erythromycin in hospital patients, mostly adults. As in previous trials, the results were to a great extent frustrated by late diagnosis. Erythromycin gave little objective benefit, but the duration of abdominal pain was less in the treated group. These results are surprising and have important implications regarding chemotherapy, for they call into question the observations of many clinicians of the benefit of erythromycin. Since the numbers of patients in the trial were too small for meaningful analysis after stratification by age and severity, care should be taken before applying these general findings to particular clinical circumstances. In other words, since erythromycin is essentially a non-toxic antibiotic, it would be wise to continue to treat moderately to severely affected patients until additional data are available. It is hoped that more trials will be run.

Plasmids

Ambrosio and Lastovica (p. 28) described a rapid screening procedure for detecting plasmids in campylobacters and reported that 21% of 350 clinical isolates (in South Africa) carried at least one plasmid. However, there was no correlation between plasmid carriage and antibiotic resistance.

A molecular analysis of tetracycline resistance (Tet R) plasmids from six strains of **C. jejuni** was the subject of a presentation by Taylor **et al.** from Canada (p. 28). Certain differences between them were shown, but they had a high degree of DNA homology. By contrast, no homology was found between these **C. jejuni** plasmids and any of the four classes of Tet R plasmids from Enterobacteriaceae.

The transmissability of Tet R plasmids was studied by Smith **et al.**, also from Canada (p. 29) and Lambert **et al.** from France (p. 30). In general, transfer was possible between closely related campylobacter species (**C. jejuni**, **C. coli**, **C. laridis** and both subspecies of **C. fetus**) but not bacteria of other genera (**Escherichia**; **Vibrio**; **Eikenella**; **Haemophilus**); the exception to this generalisation was seen in the report by Lee **et al.** (p. 30) which described the presence of campylobacter DNA in transformed **E. coli**.

M. B. Skirrow

Department of Microbiology (Pathology)
Royal Infirmary, Worcester, UK

REFERENCES

1. J. R. Warren and B. J. Marshall. Unidentified curved bacilli on gastric epithelium in active chronic gastritis. Lancet, 1983, i, 1273–1275 [letters].
2. M. Kist, K.-M. Keller, W. Niebling and W. Kilching. **Campylobacter coli** septicaemia associated with septic abortion. Infection, 1983, in press.

Abstracts of Papers Presented

A. CLINICAL ASPECTS

1. Infections due to campylobacters other than *C. jejuni* and *C. coli*

Spiral bacteria in the human stomach: a common finding in patients with gastritis and duodenal ulcer

B. J. Marshall and J. R. Warren

Departments of Gastroenterology and Pathology, Royal Perth Hospital, Perth, Australia

The human stomach is supposed to be a sterile organ with no flora of its own due to the sterilizing action of its low pH [1,2]. Since 1980 one of the authors (J.R.W.) has noted "campylobacter-like" bacteria on sections of the gastric antrum in patients with the pathological appearance of active chronic gastritis [3]. The bacteria were present in massive numbers and grew beneath the mucus, probably protected from acid. In order to determine their incidence and possible disease associations, a trial was set up and 100 consecutive gastroscopy patients consented to have antral biopsies performed. Each patient was extensively documented, and biopsy specimens were studied histologically with haemotoxylin and eosin, Warthin Starry (silver) and Gram stains, and cultured using campylobacter isolation methods. Results were as follows:

(1) Of 100 biopsy specimens, 57 contained the bacteria on Warthin Starry stain.

(2) Of those patients with gastritis 55 of 69 had the bacteria, whereas of those with normal biopsies only two of 31 had the bacteria (bacteria correlates with gastritis; $P < 0.0001$).

(3) Of 13 patients with duodenal ulcers, 13 had the bacteria (bacteria correlates with duodenal ulcer; $P = 0.001$).

(4) The bacteria were cultured in 12 cases. The bacteria are "S" shaped, 3000 nm curved rods, similar to **Campylobacter jejuni** on Gram stains. They are microaerophilic and grow up in 3 days on moist chocolate agar. Electron microscopy shows them to have up to four unipolar sheathed flagella. Most strains isolated were oxidase +, catalase +, motile, nitrate −, H_2S +, indole −, grew only at 37°C, and were resistant to nalidixic acid, but sensitive to penicillin, tetracycline, erythromycin, kanamycin, gentamicin and metronidazole.

Since these bacteria are so common and found in such numbers, their existence makes all previous treatises on gastric microbiology obsolete. Their association with gastritis and duodenal ulcer warrants further investigation.

REFERENCES

1. A. S. Freedburg and L. E. Barron. The presence of spirochetes in the human gastric mucosa. American Journal of Digestive Diseases, 1940, 7, 443-445.
2. B. S. Draser and M. J. Hudson. Spiral organisms in intestinal disease. In: Recent Advances in Infection, Vol. 1 (Edited by D. Reeves and A. Geddes). Churchill Livingstone, Edinburgh, 1979, pp. 41-53.
3. J. R. Warren and B. J. Marshall. Unidentified curved bacilli on gastric epithelium in active chronic gastritis. Lancet, 1983, i, 1273-1275 [letters].

Campylobacter fetus – twelve human isolates. Some clinical and bacteriological data

I. Heinzer

Institute of Medical Microbiology, University of Bern, Friedbuhlstrasse 51, CH-3010 Bern, Switzerland

During a 3.5 year period (September 1979 to February 1983) we isolated **Campylobacter jejuni** from 214 patients and **C. fetus** from 12 patients. In all cases **C. fetus** was found in one or more faecal samples, but blood cultures were positive in only three cases. Only three patients had an underlying disease (diabetes, chronic renal failure, leukaemia). In most cases the clinical picture was febrile enteritis, entirely similar to an infection due to **C. jejuni**. Clinical and serological data are presented.

Several selective media for campylobacters have been described in the last few years, but comparisons of these media have been reported only for **C. jejuni**. We therefore compared the ability of Butzler's, Skirrow's, Blaser's, Campy-BAP, and Preston medium to support the growth of our **C. fetus** strains. Skirrow's medium gave the best results. Campy-BAP seems to be unsuitable for the isolation of **C. fetus**.

We believe that low isolation rates for **C. fetus** in our and other laboratories are mainly caused by poor isolation techniques. Routine methods for campylobacter should also include appropriate incubation temperature and media for **C. fetus**.

2. Infections due to **C. jejuni** and **C. coli**

Studies of Campylobacter jejuni infection in volunteers

R. E. Black, M. M. Levine, M. J. Blaser, M. L. Clements and T. P. Hughes

Center for Vaccine Development, University of Maryland School of Medicine, 20 South Greene Street, Baltimore, Maryland 21201, USA

Volunteer studies with **Campylobacter jejuni** were initiated to establish certain basic features of the infection and illness, including the number of organisms needed to cause illness, the pathogenicity of different strains of **C. jejuni**, the extent of homologous and heterologous protective immunity and the nature of the immune response following infection. For these volunteer studies two strains of **C. jejuni** were used: A3004 (Penner 2) and 81-176 (Penner 23/36). To prepare the challenge inoculum 40-50 colonies of the **C. jejuni** strain were suspended in thioglycolate broth and this suspension plated onto brucella agar. After incubation overnight at 42 °C, the growth on the plate was harvested with phosphate-buffered saline and diluted to approximately the number of organisms required. Quantitative cultures were done on the inoculum before and after administration to volunteers. The inoculum was given in 150 ml of low-fat milk prepared from dry powder (except in four volunteers who were given inoculum with 2 g of sodium bicarbonate).

In dose-response studies with A3004 **C. jejuni**, 10 healthy adult volunteers ingested 8×10^2 **C. jejuni**, five become infected and one ill. Ten volunteers ingested 8×10^3 **C. jejuni**, six were infected and none ill. The rate of infection increased with increasing inocula until 100% were infected at a dose of 10^8 **C. jejuni**. The rate of ilness was 46% with 9×10^4 **C. jejuni**; however, with increasing inocula (to 10^8) the rate of illness ranged from only 9 to 22%. The average incubation to fever was 68 h and to diarrhea was 88 h. The diarrhea was mild with an average of five liquid stools and 0.5 l stool volume. In studies with strain 81-176 **C. jejuni**, three of seven volunteers given 10^6 organisms in milk developed diarrhoea; they had an average of 30 liquid stools and 2896 ml stool volume.

To document upper intestinal colonization, volunteers swallowed string devices 24 and 48 h after challenge. With 10^8 A3004 **C. jejuni**, 60% of strings were positive at 24 h and 20% at 48 h. Volunteers had blood cultures 0.5, 12, 24, 48, 72, 96 and 144 h after challenge; none of 588 cultures was positive.

Sera from volunteers before and after challenge were tested for IgM, IgG and IgA ELISA responses. Sick volunteers had an increase in all three types of antibody by day 11 after challenge; infected but non-ill volunteers also had antibody responses but of lower magnitude. Two volunteers who developed illness with 10^6 A3004 **C. jejuni** were rechallenged 1 month after recovery with 10^8 of the same strain along with five controls; neither of the **C. jejuni** veterans became infected compared with all five controls. Studies are under way to evaluate the local immune response to **C. jejuni** and the extent of homologous and heterologous protection.

Clinical features of a large outbreak of milk-borne campylobacter enteritis in a boys' boarding school

T. Hoskins* and J. R. Davies†

*Christ's Hospital, Horsham, Sussex, UK, and †Public Health Laboratory Service, 61 Colindale Avenue, London NW9 5EQ, UK

EPIDEMIOLOGY In March 1982 there was an outbreak of campylobacter enteritis in a boarding school of 785 boys between the ages of 11 and 18 years. The school is supplied with milk from its own herd, pasteurised in the dairy and distributed daily to the kitchens and boarding houses in 3-gallon and 5-gallon plastic containers. An accidental delivery of unpasteurised milk is believed to have caused the outbreak.

On 14–15 March, 10 visitors from another school stayed for 24 h and none became ill after the visit. On 15 March, three boys were admitted to the school infirmary with abdominal pain and fever. On 16 March the 14 admissions included the first cases of diarrhoea, and the outbreak reached a peak on 17 March, with 45 admissions. The milk supply from the school dairy was discontinued on 19 March, but the outbreak was already waning, with only two admissions during the weekend of 20–21 March. Of the remaining eight admissions, on 22 and 23 March, only one boy had had symptoms for less than 24 h. Confirmation that milk was the source of the infection was subsequently obtained by bacteriological studies and a questionnaire completed on 20 March by every boy in the school. Details are given by Wilson **et al.** (see abstract on p. 143).

Twelve boys present during the outbreak were known to have been infected with a different strain of campylobacter in a small outbreak in May 1980. Ten of these boys were again infected in the 1982 outbreak, eight of them reporting diarrhoea.

CLINICAL Altogether 189 boys (24.1%) reported to the infirmary with gastrointestinal symptoms, and they were evenly distributed between all 16 boarding houses and all ages. Of the 102 admitted to the infirmary all but one had fever between 37.2°C and 40.0°C. The remaining 87 had no fever at the time they were seen by the doctor or nurse. Abdominal pain, reported by 105 boys (55.6%), commonly preceded diarrhoea, which was reported by 156 (82.1%). Only one reported blood in the stools. Vomiting was reported by only 13 boys (9.4%); seven of these presented on or after 20 March, and their vomiting may have been unrelated to campylobacter infection.

CLINICAL COMPLICATIONS Between 19 and 24 March, 12 boys – not all of whom had been ill with enteritis – presented with urticaria, compared with an average number of new cases of urticaria of three per annum. No cases of reactive arthritis or erythema nodosum were seen.

Campylobacter jejuni enterocolitis in travellers' diarrhoea in Bangladesh

P. Speelman, M. J. Struelens, S. C. Sanyal and R. I. Glass

International Centre for Diarrhoeal Disease Research – Bangladesh, GPO Box 128, Dhaka-2, Bangladesh

In order to evaluate the significance of **Campylobacter jejuni** infections among travellers and expatriate residents in Bangladesh, we cultured stool specimens from 269 diarrhoeal and 196 healthy expatriates. **C. jejuni** was isolated from 45 patients with diarrhoea (17%), in 41 of whom **C. jejuni** was the sole enteropathogen (15%). Four healthy expatriates had a positive stool culture for **C. jejuni** (2%), which contrasts with considerably higher isolation rates among asymptomatic Bangladeshis.

Patients with diarrhoea associated with **C. jejuni** developed their illness earlier after arrival in Bangladesh than patients with diarrhoea of other aetiology. The onset of illness was sudden and often associated with abdominal pain (89%), fever (65%) and nausea or vomiting (43%). Half of the patients complained of myalgias and headache; 38% had faecal leukocytes and erythrocytes on microscopic examination.

Complaints of fever, abdominal cramps, dysentery, nausea or vomiting and the presence of faecal leukocytes were significantly more common in patients with **C. jejuni** and patients with **Shigella** spp. than in other diarrhoeal patients. However, infections with **C. jejuni** were less frequently associated with dysentery than infections with **Shigella** spp.

These findings indicate that **C. jejuni** is a frequent cause of travellers' diarrhoea in Bangladesh and may produce a clinical picture similar to shigellosis. The high case-to-infection ratio in expatriates and the early onset of illness after arrival may indicate the development of protective immunity.

Epidemiological studies on Campylobacter jejuni infections among infants and young children in Soweto

N. J. Richardson,* **H. J. Koornhof**,* J. L. Richardson,* P. C. B. Turnbull,* E. M. Sutcliffe,† D. M. Jones† and S. Lauwers§

*South African Institute for Medical Research, Hospital Street, Johannesburg 2000, South Africa; †Public Health Laboratory, Withington Hospital, Manchester M20 8LR, UK; and §Department of Clinical Microbiology, Free University, Brussels, Belgium

Intestinal **Campylobacter jejuni** infections are common in young children in Soweto and **C. jejuni** can frequently be recovered from faeces long after an episode of diarrhoea. The recent availability of serotyping systems prompted us to investigate the nature of long-term excretion in these children more extensively. Of 35 patients (newborn to 3 years of age) with **C. jejuni**-associated diarrhoea, 23 yielded **C. jejuni** on more than one occasion when faeces were examined at weekly intervals. Serotyping showed that some re-isolations represented true persisting excretion of the same serotype and in two instances this lasted up to 13 weeks. Strains of different serotypes were also isolated from several children examined over a period of 6 weeks. These isolations probably represent sequential infections, although mixed infections with different serotypes may have been missed as a result of the limited number of colonies picked for serotyping. In addition to **C. jejuni**, some children excreted salmonellae, shigellae and enteropathogenic **Escherichia coli** serotypes for varying periods.

Evidence of spread of **C. jejuni** serotypes was obtained in follow-up studies of families of **C. jejuni**-infected infants. In one family, there was prolonged excretion of a single serotype in the index case (3 months old) and the same serotype was subsequently isolated from two other family members (ages 3 and 32 months respectively). The older of these two children excreted at least four different **C. jejuni** serotypes over the ensuing 7 months. These studies provide clear evidence of both re-infection and prolonged excretion of **C. jejuni** in Sowetan children.

Campylobacter bacteraemia in children

D. Hanslo, T. Fryer and E. Le Roux

Department of Microbiology, Red Cross Children's Hospital, Rondebosch, Cape Town 7700, South Africa

Campylobacters are the commonest stool pathogens isolated at our hospital; they are found in 14% of patients with diarrhoea and in 3% of those without. Over the past 5 years, 63 cases of campylobacter bacteraemia have also been identified.

Blood was cultured in Castaneda-type biphasic media, growth usually being detected after 5–10 days' incubation. No particular serotype could be implicated. Of strains that were biotyped, the majority were **Campylobacter jejuni** biotype 1, but the proportion of **C. coli** was higher than is found in stool isolates.

Patients ranged in age from 2 weeks to 6 years, three-quarters being under the age of 1 year. Sexes were equally distributed. Diarrhoea was the commonest presenting complaint, occurring in 70% of cases. In less than half of these, however, could a campylobacter be isolated from the stool. Respiratory infection and convulsions accounted for a quarter of clinical presentations. Half of the patients were underweight or clinically malnourished, but only nine had a debilitating underlying illness.

Treatment was generally given before isolation of the organism, and only 70% received "appropriate" antimicrobial therapy. There was, however, little correlation between therapy and clinical progress. Two-thirds of the patients recovered promptly, including the majority of those who had not had appropriate therapy, while 34% of the patients receiving an appropriate antibiotic had a prolonged course. Four deaths occurred; in three of these patients there was severe underlying disease.

Penetration of the intestinal wall during a diarrhoeal episode seems a likely mode of pathogenesis in most, but not all, of our patients. Bacteraemia appears to be often transient, with spontaneous recovery. Further investigation of biotype or virulence factors may help to elucidate the pathogenesis of bloodstream invasion.

Clinical and epidemiological features of Campylobacter jejuni infections in Rwanda

P. De Mol and I. Habyaremye

Hopital Universitaire, Butare, Rwanda

The presence of **Campylobacter jejuni** was investigated systematically in 412 patients suffering from acute diarrhoea (of less than 4 days duration) who attended two dispensaries in the Butare area (Republic of Rwanda) during a period of 8 months. Control patients of the same age groups and socioeconomic circumstances were investigated simultaneously. **C. jejuni** was isolated from 12.6% of patients with diarrhoea but in less that 5% of the patients without diarrhoea.

The organism had a higher incidence during the dry season and the beginning of the rainy season (22%), but a lower incidence during the rainy season itself (3%). Distribution of the isolations according to age showed that infants less than 12 months old were most frequently infected (25% of all cases); the infection was relatively rare in children older than 15 years. Whatever the age group, **C. jejuni** was always isolated significantly more often from patients with diarrhoea than from others.

A systematic comparison of the symptoms and clinical findings of 83 outpatients suffering from **C. jejuni** diarrhoea with a group of patients with diarrhoea not associated with **C. jejuni** (matched for age and time of visit) showed no significant differences, except for a higher body temperature in the **C. jejuni** group; thus the clinical features of **C. jejuni** enteritis (including the presence of blood in the stools) were not distinctive.

Environmental studies showed that many domestic animals, in particular swine, were infected with **C. jejuni**, but **C. jejuni** was not found in domestic flies.

To conclude: In Rwanda, **C. jejuni** is a common cause of uncomplicated diarrhoea in children during the first years of life. In contrast to other bacterial infections controllable by environmental and water supply improvements, **C. jejuni** infections seem more difficult to limit since they are more closely related to the numerous domestic animals that are such a feature of the traditional rural way of life.

The occurrence of multiple serotypes in Campylobacter jejuni/coli enteritis

S. Lauwers and M. De Vuyst

Infectious Diseases Unit, Free University of Brussels, Brussels, Belgium

We investigated the occurrence of multiple infections in **C. jejuni** enteritis. If this phenomenon is indeed common, it must be taken into account in epidemiological studies.

All strains isolated from 177 patients - mostly children - with **C. jejuni** enteritis, from whom campylobacters had been isolated from at least two different stool samples, were serotyped by the passive haemagglutination technique using heat-stable antigens, as previously described. Altogether 481 strains were serotyped.

In a first group of 164 patients the time interval between two consecutive **C. jejuni** isolations did not exceed 14 days; in most cases the samples were taken 1 or 2 days apart. Some 32 different serotypes were encountered in this group, the serotypes LAU 1, 25, 2, 4, 5/8 and PEN 25 being the most frequent ones. In 143 patients (87.2%) all available strains from each patient belonged to the same serotype; in the remaining 21 patients (12.8%) two different serotypes were isolated from different stool samples. In three of these cases biotyping results confirmed the presence of two different strains. Although these results do not prove the occurrence of multi-serotype infections, it is likely that 12.8% of our patients harboured two different serotypes.

In a second group of 13 patients the time interval between two consecutive campylobacter isolations was at least 1 month, the longest interval being 17 months. In none of these 13 patients was the same serotype recovered during different episodes, suggesting a re-infection with another strain in all cases. Two patients experienced three episodes of **C. jejuni** enteritis, each 1-4 months apart and caused by three different serotypes.

We attempted to confirm the occurrence of multi-serotype infections by selecting at least five different colonies (typed separately) from the primary culture plate in new cases of **C. jejuni** enteritis. Until now, 22 patients have been studied, but in each of them only one serotype was found.

In conclusion, although consecutive infections with different serotypes seem to occur regularly, we could not prove the presence of multiple serotypes during a single infectious episode of campylobacter enteritis.

Endoscopic features of campylobacter colitis in children

P. Rodesch,* P. De Mol,† C. de Prez§ and S. Cadranel*

*Paediatric Gastroenterology Unit, †Microbiology and §Pathology Departments, Free University of Brussels, St Pierre Hospital, 322 rue Haute, 1000 Brussels, Belgium

Since 1976, partial or total colonoscopy, performed as soon as possible after admission, was used as an appraisal of invasiveness in 153 children with acute infective colitis. Prospective data were available from 1980 for 134 children aged 4 days to 10 years (mean 1.6 years). No complications were recorded.

Endoscopic appearances and pathological findings (graded from I to III according to the severity of the lesions) were correlated with the results of colonic biopsy and stool cultures. Culture results were as follows: salmonellas 32%, shigellas 21%, campylobacters 19%, yersinia 7%, and unidentified 21%.

In campylobacter colitis the endoscopic lesions ranged from mucosal oedema and hyperaemia with loss of the vascular pattern to disseminated groups of micro-ulcers and large confluent extensive ulceration. Pathological studies showed inter- (and sometimes intra-) glandular epithelial infiltration with a majority of polymorphonuclear cells; sometimes crypt-abscesses were also noticed. This pattern is unusual in salmonella and shigella infections where lymphocyte infiltration is predominant.

The biopsy specimens were culture positive in an average of 70% of all infected patients; however, in those infected with campylobacters, they were culture positive in only 20% of cases. Endoscopic appearances are not pathognomonic, but endoscopy is a useful, quick and reliable procedure for assessing the extent and severity of disease and thus for guiding therapy.

Post-mortem findings in six cases of fatal campylobacter infection in Bangladesh

T. Butler, M. Islam, R. Islam, P. Speelman and A. Azad

International Centre for Diarrhoeal Disease Research - Bangladesh, GPO Box 128, Dhaka-2, Bangladesh

In order to define the intestinal pathology of **Campylobacter jejuni** infection in developing countries, six fatal cases underwent post-mortem examination. All were children ranging from 1 to 10 years old. **C. jejuni** was the only enteropathogen identified in two cases; it was mixed with **Entamoeba histolytica** in two cases, with **Shigella flexneri** in one case and with **Clostridium perfringens** in one case.

In two cases characteristic lesions attributable to **C. jejuni** were observed: in the small bowel shallow and deep ulcers with mononuclear cell infiltration in the submucosa were present together with crypt abscesses; in one case there were deep ulcers in the colon which extended through the muscularis mucosae and which were surrounded by polymorphonuclear cells. In one case with **C. jejuni** as the only enteropathogen, mild inflammatory changes were present in the small bowel.

Immediate causes of death in these six cases were judged to be acute pneumonia in four cases, marasmus and shigellosis in one case, and amoebiasis in one case. Therefore, in children in Bangladesh, **C. jejuni** may contribute to death in some cases by producing inflammatory and ulcerative lesions in the small and large bowel, but in the majority of fatal cases **C. jejuni** was mixed with and probably dominated by other pathogenic agents.

A serodiagnosic study of campylobacter infection in 450 children with suspected appendicitis

A. D. Pearson, J. R. Knott, W. G. Suckling, A. C. Tuck and A. MacIver

Public Health Laboratory, Southampton General Hospital, Southampton, UK

INTRODUCTION The Southampton appendicitis project was based on the following hypotheses: firstly, appendicitis in children has multiple aetiologies; secondly, the inflammatory response seen at operation or in section may result from obstruction caused by or associated with the presence of lymphoid hyperplasia; thirdly, lymphoid hyperplasia may itself result from infection or antigenic stimulation.

PRELIMINARY INVESTIGATION **Campylobacter jejuni** was isolated from the appendix tissue, rectal swabs or peritoneal fluid in six of 251 children (2.4%) admitted to Southampton General Hospital with abdominal pain. Three children had acute appendicitis; the other three had mesenteric adenitis. Two of the mesenteric adenitis cases developed campylobacter enteritis after their discharge from hospital. The significance of campylobacters in appendicitis and mesenteric adenitis and as a cause of abdominal pain in the absence of diarrhoea has not been proven. A prospective study was designed in an attempt to establish whether there was evidence of recent or concurrent infection with gastrointestinal pathogens in children admitted to hospital with abdominal pain. This paper reports the results of **C. jejuni** antibody detection in children admitted to hospital with abdominal pain.

PROTOCOL FOR THE APPENDICITIS STUDY The survey protocol aimed to identify all children admitted to the Paediatric Department of the Southampton General Hospital between 25 April 1977 and 31 March 1979 for a period of 48 h or longer. Children with urinary tract infections or other pathologies were excluded. The clinical history, surgical findings and histology were systematised on questionnaires. Throat and rectal swabs were taken prior to surgery and blood samples for culture and serology. A peritoneal swab and the middle third of the appendix were cultured immediately after the appendicectomy. The children had a second blood test 1 month after discharge from the hospital. Antibody levels were determined for IgG to **C. jejuni/coli** (by ELISA) for streptococcal infection by ASO, DNA, MAP and ART, rotavirus by CFT to NCDV and "O" agent and by RIA for Norwalk agent. This presentation reports the results of antibody tests on 457 children admitted with abdominal pain and compares them with 324 age-matched controls. The abdominal pain group was further divided on the basis of operative findings and histology into 178 children with acute appendicitis, 12 with acute mesenteric adenitis and seven with other diagnoses. Some 191 children were admitted with abdominal pain who did not proceed to appendicectomy. The latter group was complemented with 88 children whose appendices were normal at histopathology, giving a total of 279 children in the abdominal pain group.

VALIDATION OF THE ELISA TEST The levels of IgG to **C. jejuni/coli** detected in isolate proven cases of campylobacter enteritis were $\geq$ 200 in 67 of 94 (71%) and were $\geq$ 400 in 59 of 94 (63%). These results were significantly different from the prevalence and levels of campylobacter antibody in 378 sera from antenatal patients and people with diarrhoea from whom campylobacter was not isolated.

RESULTS A total of 178 children with acute appendicitis had significantly ($P < 0.001$) higher levels and prevalence of IgG to **C. jejuni/coli** as compared to the findings in 296 age-matched controls. Some 56 of 274 (32%) had levels of IgG to **C. jejuni/coli** $\geq$ 200 and 37 of 155 (24%) had levels $\geq$ 400. A total of 279 children with abdominal pain had significantly ($P < 0.001$) higher levels and prevalence of IgG to **C. jejuni/coli** than that found in the 296 control sera. Some 68 of 242 (28%) had levels $\geq$ 200 whilst 51 of 225 (23%) had values $\geq$ 400. Comparison of the titre values in paired sera from appendicitis cases showed that 13 of 152 (9%) children had rising titres and four of 152 (3%) had falling titres, whereas in the abdominal pain group there were two of 66 (3%) with rises and two of 66 (3%) with falling titres.

HYPOTHESES (1) Campylobacter is an aetiological factor in abdominal pain in children. (2) Infection with **C. jejuni/coli** may be a predisposing or causative factor in children with acute appendicitis.

PROPOSED ACTION Undertake a double-blind trial of erythromycin in children with abdominal pain and appendicitis having first established the criteria for appendicectomy.

Campylobacter enteritis in normal and immunodeficient children

I. Melamed, Y. Bujanover, Y. Igra, D. Schwartz, V. Zakut and Z. Spirer

Paediatric Department, Rokach (Hadassah) Hospital, PO Box 51, Tel Aviv 61000, Israel

Campylobacter jejuni has recently been recognised as a common pathogen in bacterial gastroenteritis in children. During a period of 16 months, 201 cases of shigella, 56 cases of salmonella and 51 cases of campylobacter gastroenteritis were diagnosed. Five children of the campylobacter gastroenteritis group were previously known to be immunodeficient: two showed X-linked agammaglobulinemia, one had agammaglobulinemia, one had combined immunodeficiency, and one transient hypogammaglobulinemia. The average duration of fever and diarrhoea was longer in the five immunodeficient (15 and 23 days respectively) as compared with the normal children (4 and 5 days respectively). Excretion of **C. jejuni** in the stools persisted for 20-27 days in four of the immunodeficient children and for 1 year in the fifth, whereas normal children excreted **C. jejuni** for 4-16 days (average 10 days). None of the normal children had additional enteric pathogens isolated at the time of the disease, whereas four of the five immunodeficient children had shigella, salmonella or both isolated from stools at some time during the disease.

C. jejuni may be added to the list of bacterial pathogens most likely to infect immune-deficient children, especially those with a defect of the humoral system.

Clinical features of Campylobacter jejuni diarrhoea with special reference to the neonate

A. C. Velasco, M. I. Barrio, M. F. Pedreira and F. Omenaca

Servicio de Microbiologia, CSSS "La Paz", Paseo de la Castellana 261, Madrid 34, Spain

A total of 280 patients with **Campylobacter jejuni** diarrhoea were seen in a 2 year prospective study. Ages ranged from 1 day to 73 years; there were 260 children under 14 years old (10 under 1 week) and 20 adults. The sex ratio (male:female) was 1.5:1. The main clinical findings included abrupt onset of symptoms, six to seven foul odour loose stools with mucus and/or macroscopic blood. Fever and abdominal pain were frequent, but there was only occasional vomiting (10%). Rectorrhagia (as the only symptom) and convulsions were seen in two cases.

Fifty-nine patients (21%) had an underlying disease, most frequently protein intolerance and primary or acquired immunosuppression. In 28 patients (10%), other enteric pathogens were found simultaneously with **C. jejuni**.

The organism persisted in the stools for up to 8 weeks in untreated patients (3 weeks average), but could no longer be isolated after 2 days of erythromycin therapy, except in one case with a strain resistant to this drug (detected 72 h after the start of therapy).

C. jejuni is recognised as a common cause of diarrhoea at all ages; however, there are only a few reports involving neonates.

The symptoms of diarrhoea in neonates seem to be milder than those recorded in children and adults [1], except that, in our cases, blood or mucus were always present in the stools; jaundice in neonates was a prominent feature too. Only two out of the eight neonates with jaundice had anti-A isoimmunization.

Chronic diarrhoea [2] was seen in two patients, with short periods of recovery; both were cured after erythromycin therapy.

We were unable to determine whether two consecutive episodes of diarrhoea were due to reinfection or just to relapse following a period of apparently negative stool cultures [3].

Stool cultures were performed in seven mothers of infected newborns but only one yielded **C. jejuni**; she had diarrhoea some weeks before delivery. Abdominal pain, very common in adults, is difficult to evaluate in the newborn, infants and children, but usually physical findings did not suggest severe pain in the neonate. Breast feeding was continued when possible (10 cases), with good recovery without antibiotic therapy.

Strong evidence of person to person spread was detected in several hospitalised children, including two neonates.

A large number of patients presented an underlying disease, but this could just reflect an increased rate of stool cultures performed on these subjects.

SUMMARY **C. jejuni** diarrhoea lasts for an average duration of 4 days with six to seven daily stools. Boys were more frequently infected than girls, but this ratio was inverted in adults. There was a significant relationship between the number of daily stools and the presence of blood in the faeces. The clinical course of **C. jejuni** diarrhoea in neonates seemed to be milder than in children and adults, but they passed bloody and/or mucoid stools more frequently. Jaundice, with no other obvious cause, was a common feature, too, in neonates. Breast feeding should be continued whenever possible.

REFERENCES

1. G. E. Buck, M. T. Kelly, A. M. Pichanick and T. G. Pollard. **Campylobacter jejuni** in newborns: a cause of asymptomatic bloody diarrhoea. American Journal of Diseases of Childhood, 1982, **136**, 744.
2. J. R. Smalley, W. J. Klish, M. R. Brown and M. A. Campbell. Chronic diarrhoea associated with **Campylobacter**. Clinics in Paediatrics, 1982, **21**, 220.
3. V. D. Bokkenheuser and N. J. Richardson. Long term infection with **Campylobacter jejuni**. In: Campylobacter: Epidemiology, Pathogenesis and Biochemistry (D. G. Newell, ed.), PHLS, London, 1982, p. 137.

Campylobacter enteritis: a cause of failure to thrive in an infant

A. Guarino, G. Capano, C. Pignata,* B. De Vizia,* S. Guandalini and G. de Ritis*

Child Health and *Paediatric Clinic, 2nd School of Medicine, University of Naples, Naples, Italy

Campylobacter jejuni has, in the last few years, been responsible for many cases of acute enteritis, but the full spectrum of disease caused by campylobacters in childhood has not yet been thoroughly worked out. Failure to thrive was described in a child in whose stools **C. jejuni** was found associated with giardia [1].

We report a case of a 22 month old child who began having recurrent diarrhoea when she was 7 months old; her weight, despite numerous dietetic trials, including lactose-free diet, fell below the 5th percentile.

Carbohydrate malabsorption was demonstrated by the oral lactose tolerance test, but absorption of D-xylose was normal.

The more common causes of chronic diarrhoea were ruled out and **C. jejuni** was found in a stool culture. Specific serum antibodies were present at a titre of 1/160. A jejunal biopsy, performed in order to investigate the possibility of coeliac disease, revealed a jejunitis.

After oral treatment with erythromycin, the diarrhoea ceased and her weight gained rapidly, reaching, after 2 months of normal diet, the 10th percentile. Repeated stool cultures, performed after treatment, were consistently negative.

C. jejuni should be considered among the causes of failure to thrive in infancy.

REFERENCE

1. S. Cadranel, P. Rodesch, J. P. Butzler and P. Dekeyser. Enteritis due to "related vibrio" in children. American Journal of Diseases of childhood, 1973, **126**, 152–155.

B. THERAPEUTIC ASPECTS

1. Antimicrobial sensitivities and sensitivity testing

Electron-microscopic evaluation of the bactericidal activity of erythromycin on Campylobacter jejuni

R. Vanhoof,* G. Verhaegen,* D. Dekegel* and J. P. Butzler†

*Instituut Pasteur, Stoomslepersstraat 28, 1040 Brussels, and †Department of Microbiology, St Pieters Ziekenhuis, Brussels, Belgium

The aim of the study was to evaluate the bactericidal activity of erythromycin on **Campylobacter jejuni**. Susceptible and resistant strains were investigated. Growth curves of the different strains were determined. The MIC and MBC of the strains were determined by using a Cooke Dyantech MIC 2000 apparatus.

Log-phase cultures of bacteria were incubated in different concentrations of erythromycin (0.5 MIC, 1 MIC, 2 MIC, 5 MIC and 10 MIC) for various periods of time (1 h, 2 h, 4 h, 8 h, 12 h, 24 h and 32 h) and then compared with control cultures by means of transmission and scanning electron microscopy.

Serotype and biotype distribution of erythromycin and tetracycline resistant isolates of Campylobacter jejuni in Israel

J. Michel* and M. Rogol†

*Department of Clinical Microbiology, Hadassah University Hospital, Mt Scopus and †National Centre for Campylobacter, Government Central Laboratories, Ministry of Health, Jerusalem, Israel

A total of 163 isolates of **Campylobacter jejuni** were tested for their susceptibility to erythromycin and tetracycline by the agar dilution technique. They were isolated from stool samples taken from different patients during 1982. Epidemic strains were not included in this study. Serotyping of the isolates was performed by slide agglutination according to the scheme developed at the Centre for Campylobacter, Ministry of Health, Jerusalem. Biotyping was performed according to Skirrow's scheme.

Erythromycin resistance (MIC $\geq$ 8 mg/l) was observed in 24 isolates (14.7%) and tetracycline resistance (MIC $\geq$ 12 mg/l) in 67 (41.1%); 11 isolates (6.7%) were resistant to both drugs.

The isolates belonged to 54 serotypes, but the eight most frequent serotypes (11; 12; 8,23; 10; 13; 23; 4 and 26,29) represented more than 50% of all isolates. Erythromycin resistance was observed in nine serotypes and tetracycline resistance in 27. Erythromycin resistance was found to be significantly associated with serotype 12 ($P < 0.001$): over 70% of the isolates belonging to this serotype were resistant to erythromycin and it represented 50% of all isolates resistant to this drug. There was no time or geographical relationship between these resistant isolates.

The biotype distribution of the isolates showed that 83.3% belonged to biotype 1, 7.3% to biotype 2, and 9.4% were **C. coli**. Erythromycin and/or tetracycline resistance were not associated with a particular biotype. However, tetracycline resistance was more frequent in **C. coli** (61.1%), but not at a statistically significant level ($P < 0.1$).

Comparison of antimicrobial susceptibility patterns between Campylobacter jejuni and Campylobacter coli

W.-L. L. Wang, L. B. Reller and M. J. Blaser

Veterans Administration Medical Center and University of Colorado School of Medicine, Denver, Colorado, USA

In order to determine whether antibiograms are useful for separating **Campylobacter jejuni** and **C. coli**, we determined the minimum inhibitory concentrations (MICs) of 12 antibiotics for 104 human clinical strains and 74 swine strains. The standard agar dilution method (WHO-ICS) was used for the MIC tests. After preliminary testing for optimal conditions, we determined all MICs at 35 °C in an atmosphere of 5% O_2 and 10% CO_2 with 48 h of incubation. The 12 antimicrobials tested were ampicillin, amoxycillin, clindamycin, chloramphenicol, erythromycin, furazolidone, norfloxacin, nalidixic acid, rosoxacin, rosaramicin, tetracycline and Sch 32063.

Swine strains had higher MICs for four antibiotics (clindamycin, erythromycin, rosaramicin and Sch 32063) than did human strains. The differences in MICs between human and swine strains were as follows: clindamycin ($\leq$ 2 mg/l) 96% human vs 8% swine ($P < 0.001$); erythromycin ($\leq$ 8 mg/l) 96% human vs 26% swine ($P < 0.001$); rosaramicin ($\leq$ 2 mg/l) 96% human vs 21% swine ($P < 0.001$), and Sch 32063 ($\leq$ 2 mg/l) 96% human vs 8% swine ($P < 0.001$). Five of 74 (7%) swine strains were hippurate positive as were 93 of 104 (89%) human strains. Three of 11 (27%) human hippurate-negative strains were resistant to clindamycin, erythromycin, rosaramicin and Sch 32063 compared with one of 93 (1%) hippurate-positive strains. Almost all human and swine strains were susceptible to furazolidone ($\leq$ 1 mg/l) and nalidixic acid ($\leq$ 16 mg/l).

We conclude that campylobacters isolated from humans and swine have different antibiograms and that the susceptibility to certain antibiotics, such as clindamycin, may be helpful for differentiation of **C. jejuni** and **C. coli**.

The activity of seven quinoline derivatives against clinical isolates of Campylobacter jejuni

D. Felmingham, R. A. Wall and **M. D. O'Hare**

Department of Clinical Microbiology, University College Hospital, Gower Street, London WC1E 6AU, UK

The minimum inhibitory concentrations (MIC) of seven quinoline antibiotics for 100 clinical isolates of **Campylobacter jejuni** were determined. Some 10^4 colony forming units of each isolate, contained in 20 ml Mueller-Hinton Broth (Oxoid), were inoculated on to the surface of Mueller-Hinton Agar (Oxoid) plates containing 10% lysed horse blood and appropriate concentrations of antibiotic. After inoculation the plates were incubated for 48 h at 37 °C in an atmosphere of 5-12% carbon dioxide and 5-15% residual oxygen (BBL CampyPak). The minimum inhibitory concentration of each antibiotic was determined as the lowest concentration of antibiotic which completely inhibited growth of the organism tested. A control strain of **C. fetus** was included. Six newly synthesised quinoline derivatives - flumequine, rosoxacin, WIN 49375, norfloxacin, DL 8280 and ciprofloxacin - all showed significantly more activity against isolates of **C. jejuni** than did nalidixic acid. The MIC_{90} of ciprofloxacin and DL 8280, the two most active of the quinolines examined, was 0.25 mg/l. The MIC_{90} of nalidixic acid was 8.0 mg/l. In spite of this considerably higher activity against **C. jejuni**, control strains of **C. fetus** included in this study were some 16-32 times more resistant to all the quinolines examined. The clinical and taxonomic implications of these results are discussed.

In vitro susceptibility of Campylobacter jejuni to seven cephalosporins

T. Rodriguez-Gonzalez, P. Valero-Guillen, F. Guirado and F. Martin-Luengo

Department of Microbiology, Faculty of Medicine, University of Murcia, Murcia, Spain

The susceptibility of 60 strains of **Campylobacter jejuni** to seven cephalosporins (cefotaxime, ceftizoxime, cefroxadine, cefmetazole, cefsulodin, ceftriaxone and ceftazidime) was studied by the agar dilution method.

Serial dilutions of each of the drugs were incorporated into Mueller-Hinton agar in order to obtain concentrations of the drugs from 0.5 to 256 mg/l.

All the strains were plated on blood agar (Blood Agar Base No. 2, Oxoid, + 5% defibrinated horse blood) and incubated at 37 °C for 48 h in anaerobic jars under reduced oxygen tension attained by evacuating two-thirds of the air and replacing the evacuated air with a gas mixture of 90% H_2 and 10% CO_2.

The inoculum of each strain was prepared by diluting a suspension in Mueller-Hinton broth and adjusting the turbidity to No. 1 on the McFarland scale. The Mueller-Hinton plates were incubated as mentioned above, and the MICs were read after 2 days incubation. The MIC was defined as the lowest concentration that showed no growth.

The seven cephalosporins studied had a low activity against **C. jejuni.** The more active drugs were cefotaxime, ceftriaxone and ceftizoxime, inhibiting 96%, 77.5% and 62% of the strains at 32 mg/l respectively. The MICs 100 were reached by ceftriaxone and cefotaxime at 64 mg/l, at 128 mg/l for ceftizoxime, at 256 mg/l for ceftazidime and at higher than 256 mg/l for the three other drugs studied.

Campylobacter: a method for routine antimicrobial susceptibility testing

J. E. Barrett, **R. L. Kaplan** and L. J. Goodman

Presbyterian-St Luke's Hospital, 1753 West Congress Parkway,
Chicago, Illinois, USA

In order to establish a useful method for routine susceptibility testing of **Campylobacter jejuni/coli** in the clinical microbiology laboratory, we compared three media (Brucella, Wilkins Chalgren and Mueller-Hinton) and four methods (agar dilution, macrobroth dilution, Kirby Bauer disk agar diffusion and a commercial microtiter system (Sceptor, BBL)). Initially five strains of **C. jejuni/coli** were used; results were compared after 24 and 48 h incubation at both 37 and 42 °C in 5% O_2, 10% CO_2 and 85% N_2. Antimicrobials tested were choramphenicol, gentamicin, tetracycline, erythromycin, nalidixic acid, nitrofurantoin, doxycycline, N-formimidoyl thienamicin and cefotaxime.

Disk agar diffusion on Mueller-Hinton with 5% sheep blood at 42 °C in an atmosphere containing 5% O_2, 10% CO_2 and 85% N_2 was the best combination tested. Using this method, zone sizes were compared to MICs obtained from a commercial microtiter system and from agar dilution for 90 human isolates from the midwestern United States. Some 93% of the results were obtained after 24 h incubation, but the remaining 7% required 48 h. Zone sizes were established above which the organisms were susceptible: chloramphenicol, 19 mm; erythromycin, 18 mm; gentamicin, 18 mm; and tetracycline, 19 mm.

In summary, disk agar diffusion (Kirby Bauer) testing of **C. jejuni/coli** is an easy to use, cost efficient method that can be applied in any laboratory.

2. Clinical trials

Double-blind placebo-controlled trial of erythromycin in the treatment of clinical campylobacter infection

B. K. Mandal and M. E. Ellis

Regional Department of Infectious Diseases and Tropical Medicine, Monsall Hospital, Manchester, UK

During a 31-month study period, diarrhoeal patients admitted to the Regional Department of Infectious Diseases, Monsall Hospital, Manchester, who proved positive for campylobacter, were assigned blindly for treatment with a 5 day course of erythromycin (1 g/day in divided doses for adults, 50 mg/kg for children), or with a matching placebo. Symptoms were monitored and stools were cultured both during and after treatment.

Of 202 patients with proven campylobacter infection admitted during the study period, 92 were symptom-free by the time of bacteriological diagnosis and 30 proved unsuitable for trial; 80 patients entered into trial of whom 72 completed the study - 35 treated with erythromycin and 37 with placebo:

	Erythromycin group (n=35)	Placebo group (n=37)
Median duration of illness before treatment (days)	5.75	4.5
Median duration of diarrhoea after treatment (days)	1.5	1.75
Median duration of pain after treatment (days)	0.5	2.0
Number of patients with campylobacters in their stools 2 days after cessation of treatment	6	14

Blood cultures were taken routinely on admission and proved positive in one patient. Thus, erythromycin lessens pain and curtails the carriage state but otherwise does not alter the natural course of the illness, which is generally a short-lived, uncomplicated one even in hospitalised patients. The rarity of bacteraemia is also highlighted by this study.

Rapid screening procedure for detection of plasmids in campylobacters

R. E. Ambrosio and A. J. Lastovica

Department of Cytogenetics, Faculty of Medicine, University of Stellenbosch, PO Box 63, Tygerberg 7505, and Department of Microbiology, Red Cross Childrens Hospital, Rondebosch 7700, South Africa

As a consequence of difficulties in the growing of suitably dense cultures of campylobacters for plasmid extraction, it was necessary to develop a rapid screening procedure which could be used in a routine diagnostic laboratory. The method utilises the denaturing of chromosomal deoxyribonucleic acid (DNA) by alkaline sodium dodecyl sulphate (SDS) at 70 °C. The cells were lysed quickly by SDS at pH 12.6 and the lysate was cleared by heat treatment. Usually 15 min at 70 °C eliminated most of the chromosomal DNA. Plasmid yields were satisfactory and plasmids isolated were suitable for restriction endonuclease digestion after one further purification step. The procedure is rapid, inexpensive and suitable for routine screening of a large number of clinical isolates. We have screened over 480 clinical campylobacter isolates and have shown that 48% carry at least one plasmid. In no case could correlation be found between the presence of plasmids and antibiotic resistance in these organisms.

Characterisation of tetracycline-resistance plasmids from Campylobacter jejuni and Campylobacter coli

D. E. Taylor, R. S. Garner and B. J. Allan

Department of Medical Microbiology, University of Alberta, Edmonton, Alberta T6G 2H7, Canada

We have examined six strains of **Campylobacter jejuni** and **C. coli** from Belgium, Canada and the USA, which were resistant to high concentrations of tetracycline (MIC > 64 mg/l). Transmissible plasmids with molecular weights of approximately 30 x 10^6 daltons were demonstrated in all six strains. Analytical ultracentrifugation was used to determine the buoyant density of plasmid DNA, and restriction enzyme digestion was used to compare the plasmids. DNA homology amongst the plasmids was investigated by Southern blot hybridisation with ^{32}P-labelled plasmid DNA.

The density of plasmid DNAs ranged from 1.691 to 1.694 g/cm^3 (31 to 33% G+C). Of 19 restriction enzymes surveyed, four enzymes (**AccI**, **BclI**, **BglII** and **PstI**) gave four to 10 fragments and thus proved suitable for comparing the plasmids. The three plasmids from Canadian isolates showed some differences in their digestion patterns, although the two plasmids of Belgian origin had identical restriction patterns. The plasmid from an

American animal isolate yielded a different fragmentation pattern to the human isolates.

Hybridisation studies indicated that the tetracycline resistance plasmids from **C. jejuni** and **C. coli** isolated from both humans and animal sources had a high degree of DNA homology. By contrast, no homology was observed between tetracycline-resistance plasmids from campylobacters and any of the four classes of tetracycline resistance determinants encoded by plasmids from Enterobacteriaceae.

Antibiotic resistance in campylobacters with special reference to the host range of the tetracycline resistance plasmid, beta-lactamase activity and streptomycin resistance

S. J. Smith, M. A. Karmali, A. Williams, D. Kovach and P. C. Fleming

Department of Bacteriology, The Hospital for Sick Children, Toronto, Ontario, Canada

"High-level" tetracycline resistance (MIC $\geq$ 64 mg/l) in clinical isolates of **Campylobacter jejuni** has previously been shown to be mediated by a 38 x 10^6 dalton transmissable plasmid (Taylor **et al.**, 1981). The "host range" of this plasmid is currently being investigated. Tetracycline resistance transfer was performed using a plate-mating method. The donor strains consisted of a tetracycline-resistant clinical isolate of **C. jejuni** (MK175) and a tetracycline-resistant **C. fetus** subsp. **fetus** transconjugant (SS-1) which had been derived from mating **C. fetus** subsp. **fetus** (ATCC 27344) with **C. jejuni** (MK175). Tetracycline resistance determinants were successfully transferred from **C. jejuni** (MK175) to **C. fetus** subsp. **fetus** (ATCC 27374), **C. fetus** subsp. **venerealis** (ATCC 19483), **C. coli** (PC66) and NARTC strain (Skirrow 299-80); and also from **C. fetus** subsp. **fetus** (SS-1) to **C. coli** and **C. jejuni**. The frequency ranged from 10^{-3} to 10^{-5} (transconjugants/recipient). Transfer was not achieved with **C. sputorum** (PC62), Group II (aerotolerant) strain (PC367), the nitrogen-fixing campylobacter (CI) and the NARTC strain (Skirrow 299-80). Transconjugants were confirmed by determining the MICs to tetracycline and by DNA plasmid isolation using a modified method of Birnboim and Doly (1979). Further attempts to transfer the resistance plasmid to **Escherichia coli** and to **Vibrio parahaemolyticus**, (PC101), **V. cholerae** (PC102), **Eikenella corrodens**, (PC112), and **Haemophilus influenzae** type b (clinical isolate) were unsuccessful.

Recent observations on the antibiotic sensitivity patterns have shown that of 28 strains of **C. fetus** subsp. **fetus** tested, all were very sensitive to erythromycin, tetracycline, chloramphenicol and gentamicin. Ampicillin MICs ranged from 0.5 to 16 mg/l, but in contrast to **C. jejuni** resistance was not associated with beta-lactamase production. Further, 64% of **C. coli** tested (77 strains tested) had MICs to streptomycin ranging from 8 to $\geq$ 512 mg/l. Some 54.6% of these strains had MICs of $\geq$ 512 mg/l. By contrast, 93% of **C. fetus** subsp. **fetus** (30 strains) and of **C. jejuni** (75 strains) tested were found to have MICs to streptomycin of $\leq$ 4 mg/l. The nature of streptomycin resistance in campylobacters is presently being investigated.

Plasmid-mediated tetracycline resistance in Campylobacter jejuni

T. L. Lambert, F. W. Goldstein, B. Papadopoulou and J. F. Acar

Laboratoire de Microbiologie, Hopital Saint Joseph, 7 rue Pierre Larousse, 75014 Paris, France

Campylobacter jejuni strains resistant to tetracycline have previously been reported from Belgium, Canada, Israel and the USA. During a 3 year period, seven out of 80 strains isolated were resistant to tetracycline; five strains were epidemiologically unrelated. The tetracycline resistance marker was transferred from six out of the seven strains to **C. fetus** and **C. jejuni**. Attempts to transfer the tetracycline resistance marker into **Escherichia coli** were unsucessful.

Plasmid analysis by gel electrophoresis suggests that resistance to tetracycline is governed by three different plasmids of respectively 24 x 10^6, 28 x 10^6 and 29 x 10^6 daltons molecular weight, which are different from the plasmids isolated in Canada.

Complementation of an auxotrophic mutation in Escherichia coli by cloned Campylobacter jejuni genes

E. C. Lee, M. E. Dobson and S. D. Stewart

Naval Medical Research Institute, Bethesda, Maryland, USA

This research is directed at the study of the genetic control of various campylobacter gene products and their role in virulence. A genomic library for a clinical **Campylobacter jejuni** isolate has been constructed by cloning fragments obtained by partial digestion of high molecular weight DNA with Sau3A into the BamH1 site of pBR322. The recombinant plasmids were used to transform **Escherichia coli** HB101; successful transformation was indicated by the normally antibiotic-sensitive HB101 displaying plasmid-mediated ampicillin resistance. Recombinant plasmids were distinguished from prototype plasmids by the recombinants' failure to confer tetracycline resistance on the host organism.

The presence of campylobacter DNA in transformed **E. coli** cells was confirmed by nucleic acid hybridization with radiolabeled campylobacter DNA. The campylobacter DNA in the recombinant plasmid, pCP1, was shown to complement an auxotrophic defect in HB101 which prevented its growth on media lacking the amino acid proline. The campylobacter DNA inserted into pBR322 coded for gamma-glutamylphosphate reductase, an enzyme lacking in HB101.

This is the first report of a campylobacter gene product synthesized in a bacterial cell of another genus. The fact that the gene product is expressed suggests that **E. coli** is able to recognize the control sequence in campylobacters.

Other recombinant plasmid containing **E. coli** clones have been isolated. We are in the process of identifying the gene products of these isolates.

Session II

TAXONOMY, BIOTYPING, ISOLATION AND DETECTION

Report on the Session

TAXONOMY AND BIOTYPING

Molecular aspects

During the 2.5 years since the First International Workshop, several taxonomic uncertainties have been resolved. **C. coli** has been shown to be a species in its own right rather than a biotype of **C. jejuni**; the principal phenotypic difference between the two is the unique ability (among campylobacters) of **C. jejuni** to hydrolyse hippurate. The NARTC group of Skirrow and Benjamin has been formally described [1] as a new species with the proposed name of **C. laridis** (Greek, **laros** = a sea bird). **C. sputorum** subsp. **mucosalis** has also been formally described and the name validated [2]. Resolution of these taxonomic uncertainties has been attained mainly through DNA analyses and hybridisation studies, which have been conveniently summarised and reviewed by Owen [3]. However, work completed after that review had been written was the subject of a presentation by Ursing **et al.** at this Workshop (p. 39).

In general Ursing's results confirmed previous work, but two new genetically distinct groups were also described. The first of these is the "CNW" (catalase negative or weak) group described by Sandstedt, Ursing and Walder [4]. These organisms were isolated from dogs in Sweden and had a DNA relatedness to **C. jejuni** and **C. coli** of about 40%. They grow more slowly than **C. jejuni** to produce a rather delicate flat spreading type of colony. Apart from their weak or negative catalase activity, they differ from **C. jejuni** in growing less well at 42 °C, failing to hydrolyse hippurate, and being at least as sensitive to cephalothin and triphenyltetrazolium chloride as **C. fetus.** A few strains of this type had also been isolated from dogs in the UK and independently recognised as a new group (M. B. Skirrow and J. Benjamin, unpublished).

The second new group described by Ursing **et al.** consisted of strains isolated from pigs and cattle and they were genetically more related to **C. fetus.** They are similar to, or perhaps even the same as, **C. hyointestinalis**, an organism also found in pigs and cattle and recently described by Gebhart **et al.** [5] (see also Chang **et al.**, p. 130).

There were two presentations on the protein profiles of **Campylobacter** spp. as detected by SDS-polyacrylamide gel electrophoresis (PAGE). Costas and Owen (p. 40) described a single major protein band for each campylobacter group. For example **C. sputorum** and **C. fecalis** each had a major band at 44,000 daltons, and **C. jejuni**, **C. coli** and **C. laridis** shared bands in the range of 39,000–41,000 daltons. Minor bands numbering 40–50 formed patterns that were often distinctive. For example serotypes B and C of **C. sputorum** subsp. **mucosalis** had a pattern that was consistently different from serotype A of the same subspecies. On the other hand, **C. jejuni** and **C. coli** showed a range of minor band patterns that did not correlate with biotype or serotype. Computer analysis is being used to improve the recognition and discrimination of patterns.

Lastovica **et al.** (p. 40) obtained somewhat different values for major protein bands. For example they reported a figure of 44,000–45,000 daltons for **C. coli** and 42,000 daltons for **C. jejuni**. But like Costas and Owen they detected a distinctive pattern of minor bands in **C. laridis.** They also suggested that two-dimensional PAGE, which could differentiate between proteins of different amino acid sequence but of the same molecular weight, would be more likely to show strain differences than one-dimensional tests.

Krausse and Ullman (p. 41) tested various **Campylobacter** spp. for the production of volatile and non-volatile fatty acids by high performance liquid chromatography (HPLC). All produced succinic, acetic and butyric acids, but **C. jejuni** and **C. coli** were the only species to produce pyruvic and/or malonic acids (**C. laridis** was not tested). None of the six **C. coli** strains tested produced malonic acid but 11 of 13 strains of **C. jejuni** did so. Only one strain of **C. jejuni** failed to produce pyruvic acid. Additional tests, notably DNAase and hydrolysis of Tween® 40, 60 and 80, were used to divide **C. jejuni** and **C. coli** into additional biotypes. **C. fecalis** was unique in producing fumaric acid, but **C. sputorum** subsp. **bubulus** (which is closely related) was not tested. **C. sputorum** subsp. **mucosalis** did not produce fumaric acid.

Biotyping

During the past two years the hippurate test has been validated. **C. jejuni** is the only member of the genus to hydrolyse hippurate, and strains capable of doing so show a high degree of genetic relatedness [3].

The test for H_2S production in a specific iron/bisulphite/pyruvate medium (FBP broth), described by Skirrow and Benjamin [6] and used by them for dividing **C. jejuni** into two biotypes, did not prove to be reliable in the hands of some workers. However, Lior's presentation at this meeting (p. 42) has now placed this simple test on a sound footing by defining more precisely the conditions necessary for its correct performance. It seems that the most important factor omitted from the original description of the test is the need to buffer the FBP medium to a pH of about 7.3. The unbuffered medium is liable to become acid on storage and this inhibits the H_2S reaction. It is necessary to grow the test organism in a reduced oxygen atmosphere (about 6%) before inoculating the FBP broth. The effect of atmosphere on H_2S production, as well as the effect of growth temperature and the presence of pyruvate, was described by Jorgensen (p. 43). Amongst other things she found that H_2S production in FBP broth was enhanced if hydrogen was present in the atmosphere during the first growth stage of the test (hydrogen is known to be an important substrate for **C. jejuni**).

Attempts to differentiate **C. jejuni** and **C. coli** according to DNAase production have hitherto not met with much success. Even the strongest producer is weak by comparison with, say, **Staphylococcus aureus**, and discrimination between positive and negative reactions is difficult. However, Lior described a modification of the test that overcomes this difficulty and he used the test to extend the biotype divisions of Skirrow and Benjamin for **C. jejuni** and to divide **C. coli** and **C. laridis** each into two biotypes. In order to avoid confusion, Roman numerals were chosen to designate the Lior biotypes (Skirrow and Benjamin used Arabic numerals) and this has the added advantage of distinguishing biotype from serotype numbers. If the DNAase test proves to be generally reproducible, the former Skirrow and Benjamin biotype numbers for **C. jejuni** will become obsolete. The relationship of the two schemes is as follows:

Skirrow	**H_2S (FBP)**	**Lior**	**DNAase**
C. jejuni biotype 1	−	**C. jejuni** biotype I	−
		C. jejuni biotype II	+
C. jejuni biotype 2	+	**C. jejuni** biotype III	−
		C. jejuni biotype IV	+

Future subdivisions will be more easily fitted into four- than two-numbered categories. Difficulties will doubtless be encountered, which makes it all the more important to encourage free discussion of any new proposals. Lior regarded biotyping as complementary to serotyping (Lior **et al.**, p. 87). His methods are shortly to be published in full.

Another approach to biotyping was displayed by Bolton **et al.** (p. 42). They chose to use a numerical coding system in the manner of API gallery tests. A set of four numbers represented patterns of biochemical, temperature, or resistance tests. For example, a set of numbers beginning with the figure "1" means that the organism grows at 25 °C and that it therefore could not be any of the thermophilic species. Similarly any set of figures beginning with "6" identifies the organism as **C. jejuni**, because a score of 6 means that hippurate was hydrolysed. Subsequent numbers code a strain within a species or group. This approach could be valuable in epidemiological studies.

Elharrif and Megraud (p. 44) screened many strains of **C. jejuni** and **C. coli** for a wide range of enzymes and ended up with an experimental API-ZYME micro-gallery of 10 selected enzymes, which included alkaline phosphatase. Differences between the reactions of **C. jejuni** and **C. coli** were found in the case of two enzymes, but the distribution of other enzymes was not related to either the species or their origin (animal or human). This is a promising line of work and we look forward to hearing more from this team in Bordeaux.

A new difference between **C. fetus** and other campylobacters was shown by Firehammer and Border (p. 44). Both subspecies of **C. fetus**, but especially **C. fetus** subsp. **fetus**, were distinctly more resistant to the bacteriostatic compound irgasan than other bacteria, including some **Proteus** spp. and other enterobacteria though not **Pseudomonas.** Irgasan may therefore not only be of value in distinguishing **C. fetus** from other campylobacters, but also as a selective agent in campylobacter isolation media.

Morphological aspects

The presentation of Skirrow **et al.** (p. 45) gave an overview of the flagellar and general morphology of most of the recognised groups of campylobacter including some new bacteria of uncertain status. A simple flagellar stain gave results that permitted measurement of both flagellar and cell wavelengths comparable to those obtained by electron microscopy. Notable findings were: (1) that **C. fetus** subsp. **venerealis** cultures contained up to 10% lophotrichate cells (up to five flagella at one pole) and tufts of lateral flagella at points of presumptive cell division; (2) that **C. fecalis** and **C. sputorum** subsp. **bubulus** had similar and distinct morphologies characterised by unusually long flagella (monotrichate) with a short wavelength relative to cell wavelength. Apart from differences in catalase activity these bacteria are phenotypically similar and are probably more closely related than has been thought.

On a quite different plane, Curry **et al.** (p. 46) showed some truly remarkable electron micrographs of the flagellar attachment apparatus of **C. jejuni.** The dish-like discs they describe in their abstract were shown to have 11 spokes or segments which gave them the appearance of a cartwheel. They were able to demonstrate this by a process of repeated photographic imaging with incremental rotation. Apparently nothing quite like these structures has been seen before; they may be peculiar to campylobacters and therefore of taxonomic significance. Studies of **Spirillum** spp. showed somewhat similar disc-like structures but without any segmentation.

Newly described campylobacters and campylobacter-like organisms

The wider use of endoscopy and the opportunity to obtain mucosal specimens has given a new perspective to the study of the gut flora. As a result, several new campylobacter-like organisms have been discovered. The two presentations from Seattle (Fennell **et al.**, p. 47; Totten **et al.**, p. 48) described no less than three groups of such organisms - temporarily designated CLO-1, CLO-2 and CLO-3 (one strain only) - associated with proctitis in homosexual men (see editorial comment on p. 6). Totten **et al.** showed that CLO-1 consisted of two closely related sub-groups, each containing strains showing > 90% DNA homology. These strains are somewhat similar to the CNW group isolated from dogs in Sweden [4] (see also p. 33), but side by side comparisons have not been made. CLO-2 strains also showed > 90% DNA homology within their own group, but < 10% with other campylobacter groups. In culture they were said to give off a distinctive odour likened to hypochlorite disinfectant. Examination of a representative CLO-2 strain (Skirrow **et al.**, p. 45) showed it to be rather spirochaetal in form; long and slender with an amphitrichate flagellar configuration. CLO-1 and CLO-2 strains had a DNA G+C content of 37-38 mol%, just inside the currently defined campylobacter range. The CLO-3 strain had a value of 45% and is probably not a campylobacter.

What of the spiral bacteria of Marshall and Warren (p. 11) that are found in the gastric antra of patients with peptic ulcer and gastritis (see editorial comment on p. 5)? These bacteria were initially thought to be **Spirilla** because they possess up to four polar flagella. However, the fact that a proportion of **C. fetus** subsp. **venerealis** cells have such a configuration (see above) suggests that this feature should not be exclusive to the genus **Campylobacter**. Moreover, metabolically they resemble campylobacters: they are strictly microaerophilic (exposure to atmospheric oxygen for 15 h was lethal in one experiment), they have no action on sugars, and are sensitive to metronidazole - a feature rare among non-anaerobic bacteria but shown by several groups of campylobacter. Most important, the DNA G+C content (single strain examined) was 34 mol%, which is right in the middle of the campylobacter range. As previously mentioned, their specific location and association makes the provisional name of "pyloric campylobacter" particularly apt; **pylorus** is Greek for gatekeeper - one who looks both ways. Should these bacteria prove to be campylobacters then **Campylobacter pyloridis** would be an appropriate name.

In a presentation by Neill **et al.** (p. 48) the aerotolerant campylobacters were described as a heterogenous yet clearly distinct group. This was shown by PAGE of acid-phenol protein extracts and data on whole cell fatty acid composition. The special features of this group are the ability to grow freely in air and at 15 ºC. This is un-campylobacter-like behaviour, but their DNA composition (G+C of 29-34 mol%) suggests that they do belong to this genus.

ISOLATION AND DETECTION

One method of detecting campylobacters in body tissues - an important facility for the study of pathogenesis - is by an immunofluorescent procedure. It was encouraging, therefore, to see two developments along these lines, though neither is yet at a stage where the detection of bacteria in sections can be expected. The method of Dolby **et al.** (p. 49) gave good specificity but only moderate sensitivity for the detection of **C. jejuni** in faeces. Yet campylobacters were seen lying adjacent to the mucosa in rectal biopsy specimens. Lambe and Campbell (p. 50) are developing an ELISA in the hope of increasing the sensitivity and, it seems, the specificity of detection. Antisera made against SDS-treated outer membranes appear to be capable of distinguishing between **C. jejuni** and **C. coli.** It would be fair to say that these tests are still in experimental stages. Immunoperoxidase methods may, however, be a better approach to this problem.

A novel form of culture methodology was introduced by Humphrey and Cruickshank (p. 51), who studied the effect of cold shock on the isolation of **C. jejuni**. This work has particular relevance to the isolation of **C. jejuni** from food, milk and other materials that may have been subjected to low temperatures before being sent for culture. There were some curious findings. For example, the addition of polymyxin to a culture medium protected cold-shocked bacteria from a progressive decline in numbers that occurred in plain medium, but not with all strains tested. Rifampicin had the opposite effect and was considered unsuitable for inclusion in media designed to isolated **C. jejuni** from specimens that might have been frozen or chilled.

These observations had perhaps less relevance to one major aspect of campylobacter disease, namely the problems of culturing **C. jejuni** and **C. coli** from patients in developing countries. There were two approaches. Goossens **et al.** (p. 53) used an improved medium with high selectivity and sensitivity that gave acceptable results in a simple candle extinction jar, even at 37 °C thus eliminating the need for costly gas generating kits or a dedicated incubator. The other approach, of Bolton **et al.** (p. 52), was to design a blood-free medium which would be cheaper and more convenient to prepare. The key to the success of this medium was the use of charcoal instead of blood; but this created problems by interfering with the selective agents normally used in campylobacter media - except for cephalosporins. Much work went into the design of this medium and the authors claim that it performs virtually as well as the orthodox Preston method. It remains to be seen whether it performs as well in a candle jar as in the usual campylobacter atmosphere. If it does, it will indeed be a major advance.

There were several presentations that compared more established media or assessed the value of selective enrichment culture. Enrichment is essential for the isolation of campylobacters from food and environmental samples, but whether enrichment is cost effective for the culture of faeces from ill patients is debatable. It may be more economical and as clinically effective to culture more than one sample from those patients in whom a bacteriological diagnosis is important. A 16% increase in isolation rate with multiple sampling was reported in one clinical study [7].

Steele and McDermott (p. 54) presented a particularly neat and simple method of selective culture using 450 nm membrane filters applied to non-selective media. The great advantage of the method is that it is capable of isolating strains that are unduly susceptible to antimicrobials (quite a lot according to their results), and filter holders and syringes are not required. It will probably have a useful application for the isolation of **Campylobacter** spp. that do not grow on **C. jejuni** selective media. Unfortunately the cost of the membrane filters (roughly 85p = US $1.28) prohibit their use as a routine method in developing countries.

For those who earn their living by safeguarding the fertility and welfare of bovine mothers, the presentation of Lander **et al.** (p. 56) is of great interest. Improved methods for diagnosing venereal vibriosis and detecting the carrier state in bulls were displayed with a clarity that - for non-veterinarians - verged on the alarming. The same authors reported on an ELISA technique for detecting antibodies to **C. fetus** in bovine vaginal mucus in the session on serodiagnosis (see Gill **et al.**, p. 74).

It is appropriate to conclude this section by drawing attention to the presentation by Tompkins **et al.** (p. 50), because it could have far-reaching implications for the future pattern of laboratory work. They used a specific DNA probe to detect **C. jejuni** in stools. At present the method is not particularly sensitive but it will no doubt be improved in time.

More significant is the application of an ELISA to detect the DNA probe. Such an adaptation potentially brings the technique within the reach of non-specialist laboratories without the need for costly equipment for measuring radioactivity. This is something for the future, but the prospects are fascinating.

M. B. Skirrow

Department of Microbiology (Pathology),
Royal Infirmary, Worcester, UK

REFERENCES

1. J. Benjamin, S. M. Leaper, R. J. Owen and M. B. Skirrow. Description of **Campylobacter laridis**, a new species comprising the nalidixic acid resistant thermophilic **Campylobacter** (NARTC) group. Current Microbiology, 1983, **8**, 231-238.

2. G. H. K. Lawson, J. L. Leaver, G. W. Pettigrew and A. C. Rowland. Some features of **Campylobacter sputorum** subsp. **mucosalis** subsp. nov., nom., rev., and their taxonomic significance. International Journal of Systematic Bacteriology, 1981, **31**, 385-391.

3. R. J. Owen. Nucleic acids in the classification of campylobacters. European Journal of Clinical Microbiology, 1983, **2**, 367-377.

4. K. Sandstedt, J. Ursing and M. Walder. Thermotolerant **Campylobacter** with no or weak catalase activity isolated from dogs. Current Microbiology, 1983, **8**, 209-213.

5. C. J. Gebhart, G. E. Ward, K. Chang and H. J. Kurtz. **Campylobacter hyointestinalis** (new species) isolated from swine with lesions of proliferative ileitis. American Journal of Veterinary Research, 1983, **44**, 361-367.

6. M. B. Skirrow and J. Benjamin. Differentiation of enteropathogenic campylobacter. Journal of Clinical Pathology, 1980, **33**, 1122.

7. T. Pitkanen, R. Pettersson, A. Ponka and T. U. Kosunen. Clinical and serological studies in patients with **Campylobacter fetus** spp. **jejuni** infection: I. Clincial findings. Infection, 1981, **9**, 274-278.

Abstracts of Papers Presented

A. TAXONOMY AND BIOTYPING

1. Molecular aspects

DNA homology groups of thermotolerant Campylobacter spp.

J. B. Ursing,* K. Sandstedt† and M. Walder*

*Department of Medical Microbiology, University of Lund, Malmo General Hospital, S-214 01 Malmo, and †National Veterinary Institute, Ultuna, S-750 07 Uppsala, Sweden

Thermotolerant **Campylobacter** is here defined as **Campylobacter** spp. growing at 42 °C but not at 25 °C. The strains investigated were field strains from human and animal sources and reference strains of recognised species of **Campylobacter**. G+C was estimated by thermal denaturation and DNA-DNA relatedness by the hydroxyapatite method.

Five DNA-relatedness groups of thermotolerant **Campylobacter** spp. could be recognised with an intragroup relative binding rate (RBR) of over 80% for all groups:

(1) **C. jejuni**
(2) **C. coli**
(3) **Campyl.** spp (NARTC)

These groups had G+C from 31.2 to 33.1 mol%. The relatedness between **C. jejuni** and **C. coli** was about 60%, and between these species and the NARTC group about 40%.

(4) A group of strains with negative or weak catalase activity isolated from dog faeces. These strains had a G+C content of 35.2–35.8 mol% and were about 40% related to **C. jejuni** and **C. coli**.

(5) A group of nalidixic acid resistant faecal strains isolated from pigs and cattle. Their G+C content was 35.0–35.8 mol% and their RBRs versus **C. jejuni** and **C. coli** below 20%.

Groups 4 and 5 seem to represent new campylobacters. It is possible that they will deserve species rank when their phenotypic properties have been subjected to more extensive study.

The classification and identification of campylobacters using total protein profiles

M. Costas and R. J. Owen

Central Public Health Laboratory, National Collection of Type Cultures, 175 Colindale Avenue, London NW9 5HT, UK

The total protein patterns of strains (150+) representing six species of **Campylobacter** have been examined using the technique of SDS-polyacrylamide gel electrophoresis. A single major band of protein was evident in the electrophoretograms of all **Campylobacter** strains examined. The relative mobility of this protein band could be used to separate a number of the species presently contained within the genus. For example, **C. sputorum** and **C. fecalis** were characterised by a major protein band of approximate molecular weight 44,000 daltons, whereas the **C. jejuni/coli** group and **C. laridis** possessed a band of approximate molecular weight 39,000–41,000 daltons. Strains of **C. fetus** gave a major protein band intermediate between these two groups of values at an approximate molecular weight of 42,000 daltons. In addition to this major band, the overall pattern which consisted of about 40–50 bands could also be used to distinguish clearly between many of the species. This is shown in **C. laridis** which gives a distinctive and recognisable pattern. Similarly **C. sputorum** and **C. fetus** gave distinct patterns again characteristic of the species. The problematic **C. jejuni/coli** group gave a range of patterns which did not correlate with either the simple biotyping scheme or the more complex serotyping schemes which have been proposed. Work is currently in progress on the analysis of the data using computer assisted techniques such as that devised by Jackman [1].

REFERENCE

1. P. J. H. Jackman. Classification of **Corynebacterium** species from axillary skin by numerical analysis of electrophoretic protein patterns. Journal of Medical Microbiology, 1982, 15, 485.

Protein profiles from clinical and environmental isolates of Campylobacter spp.

A. J. Lastovica,* R. Kirby,† S. Carr† and F. Robb†

*Department of Microbiology, Red Cross Hospital, and †Department of Microbiology, University of Cape Town, Rondebosch 7700, Cape Town, South Africa

We have examined over 30 clinical, avian and canine faecal isolates of **Campylobacter fetus, C. jejuni/coli** and nalidixic acid resistant thermophilic campylobacters. Concurrent testing has demonstrated enterotoxins and adhesins in some of the clinical isolates. Protein profiles were done using these isolates and their cell-free culture fluids by SDS-polyacrylamide gel electrophoresis in 10% slab gels.

Many bands were evident with similar mobilities in all the strains examined. The major outer membrane components were in the same molecular weight range in clinical as well as environmental isolates. **C. fetus** typed strains and clinical isolates all have two major protein bands (40,000 and 45,000 daltons MW) which are readily distinguishable from the **C. jejuni/coli** group. The latter have one major protein band which appears to have either 40,000 or 45,000 dalton MW. The environmental isolates closely resembled those **C. jejuni/coli** typed strains whose major band occurred at 40,000 dalton MW.

The culture supernatants of the isolates varied considerably in terms of protein concentration; however, the protein banding patterns showed relatively little variation. Out of 21 bands which could be readily distinguished, three bands showed variability between strains.

Identification of Campylobacter species using high performance liquid chromatography and biochemical tests

R. Krausse and U. Ullman

Department of Medical Microbiology of the University, University of Kiel, Brunswikerstrasse 2-6, 2300 Kiel, Federal Republic of Germany

A total of 56 non-copy strains of **Campylobacter jejuni** isolated from diarrhoeal patients were characterised by biochemical tests. The following reactions were performed: hydrolysis of hippurate, reduction of nitrite and nitrate, activity of desoxyribonuclease, and hydrolysis of Tween® 40, 60 and 80. Including the different hydrolysis of the Tweens®, 23 biotypes could be distinguished. According to lipolytic activity only, 14 biotypes were detected. Thus biotype 1 was isolated in 19.6% and biotype 2 in 16%; three biotypes were observed only once.

Of the 56 **C. jejuni** strains, 19 were analysed for the production of volatile and non-volatile fatty acid using high performance liquid chromatography (HPLC) in connection with a column for organic acids (Aminex HPX-87 H). A standard mixture of 21 short-chain fatty acids was taken as reference. By this method five biotypes could be characterised. The most frequent biotype was type 1 (52.6%). All the biotypes produced succinic acid, acetic acid and butyric acid. Differences exist in the production of pyruvic acid, malonic acid and isobutyric acid. **C. jejuni** can be distinguised clearly by HPLC technique from all the other **Campylobacter** species. No differences exist between **C. fetus** subsp. **fetus**, **C. fetus** subsp. **venerealis** and **C. sputorum** subsp. **mucosalis**. **C. fecalis**, however, can be differentiated by the production of fumaric acid.

2. Biotyping (mainly **C. jejuni**, **C. coli** and **C. laridis**)

A new extended biotyping scheme for Campylobacter jejuni, Campylobacter coli and "Campylobacter laridis" (NARTC)

H. Lior

National Enteric Reference Center, Bureau of Bacteriology, Laboratory Center for Disease Control, Tunney's Pasture, Ottawa, Ontario K1A 0L2, Canada

A biotyping scheme based on hippurate hydrolysis, DNA hydrolysis and modified FBP agar for detection of rapid H_2S production was applied to **Campylobacter jejuni** (962 cultures), **C. coli** (290 cultures) and "**C. laridis**" (16 cultures) isolated from human cases of enteritis, chickens, turkeys, cattle, swine and other animals. The results obtained with the above tests allow the recognition of the following biotypes:

C. jejuni	**C. coli**	**"C. laridis"**
Biotype I	Biotype I	Biotype I
Biotype II	Biotype II	Biotype II (?)
Biotype III		
Biotype IV		

Of the 769 **C. jejuni** isolates from human cases of enteritis, 52% belonged to biotype I, 39% to biotype II, 5% to biotype III and 4% to biotype IV. Among 193 **C. jejuni** isolates from non-human sources, 55% of 115 isolates from cattle were biotype I and 42% were biotype II. Most chicken and turkey isolates belonged to biotypes I and II. Of the 168 **C. coli** isolates from human cases of enteritis, 59% were biotype I and 41% were biotype II. Most **C. coli** isolates from chickens and turkeys belonged to biotype I while 66% of 83 isolates from fresh and sea water from the UK were biotype I and 34% belonged to biotype II. All "**C. laridis**" isolates investigated so far belonged to biotype I. The integration of the biotyping and serotyping schemes allows the subdivision of the major serogroups by biotypes. This extended biotyping system provides additional markers, thereby increasing the discriminating power of serotyping for epidemiological investigations.

Experiences with an extended biotyping scheme for Campylobacter species

F. J. Bolton, A. V. Holt and **D. N. Hutchinson**

Public Health Laboratory, Royal Infirmary, Meadow Street, Preston PD1 6PS, UK

Isolation of **Campylobacter jejuni** is now commonplace, but typing methods of epidemiological value are not widely available. Skirrow and Benjamin have described several tests which may be useful for biotyping, and their shortened scheme has become widely accepted. Unfortunately this scheme is of limited value for epidemiological investigation.

We have investigated the susceptibility of campylobacters to a selection of antibiotics, dyes and chemicals in a search to find a set of differential tests. We have modified some tests described by other workers and included several new tests. The following tests have been selected to date: (a) hippurate hydrolysis; (b) temperature tolerance, i.e. growth at 25 °C; (c) resistotyping using

cephazolin	safranin O
potassium permanganate	sodium arsenite
triphenyltetrazolium chloride	nalidixic acid
pyronin Y	5-fluorouracil
metronidazole	O-cycloserine

These tests are arranged in four groups of three tests each. A numerical coding system is then used to classify results, and this leads to a four-figure biotype code. NCTC reference strains and **C. fetus** strains have given consistently reproducible results.

This scheme has been applied epidemiologically for the typing of campylobacters from milk-borne outbreaks in the UK. Different biotypes were distinguished in unrelated outbreaks of **C. jejuni** infection within the same Penner serogroups.

This scheme speciates and biotypes campylobacters and different biotyopes can be recognised within serogroups. **C. laridis** strains are more sensitive to cephazolin than other thermophilic campylobacters, and this test has proved useful for identification of nalidixic acid-sensitive strains of **C. laridis**. The need for both biotyping and serotyping of isolates for full epidemiological value has been demonstrated.

Hydrogen sulphide production by thermophilic members of the genus Campylobacter

K. Jorgensen

Institute of Hygiene and Microbiology, Royal Veterinary and Agricultural University, Copenhagen, Denmark

A comparison of the influence of growth temperature (37 or 43 °C) and the effect of nitrogen or hydrogen in controlled growth atmospheres on the ability of thermophilic campylobacters to produce hydrogen sulphide was measured by the amount of blackening produced. Nutrient broth No. 2 (Oxoid) plus 0.12% agar was used as basal medium with varied supplement combinations of $FeSO_4.7H_2O$ (0.03/0.05%), ferric ammonium citrate (0.07%), sodium metabisulphite (0.05%), sodium pyruvate (0.05/0.5%), glucose (0.05/0.5%) and cysteine-HCl (0.05%). The test tubes were incubated aerobically at 37 and 43 °C and examined hourly (2 and 4 h) and again after 1, 3 and 5 days.

The growth and test temperatures used had no apparent influence on the amount of blackening, in contrast to the growth atmospheres. The blackening was greater and more reproducible when hydrogen was used in the atmospheres instead of nitrogen. $FeSO_4.7H_2O$ was simply a better indicator than ferric ammonium citrate. When sodium metabisulphite was present in the test media, maximum blackening appeared in a few hours, in contrast to 1-3 days for other supplement combinations. It was noted that sodium pyruvate heavily influenced the blackening, depending on the supplement combinations. The hydrogen sulphide production from cysteine-HCl could be suppressed by addition of 0.05% pyruvate and the reaction was totally inhibited by 0.5% pyruvate. In contrast to this, 0.05% or 0.5% pyruvate does not inhibit the hydrogen sulphide production from sodium metabisulphite.

Enzymatic profiles of thermophilic campylobacters

Z. Elharrif and F. Megraud

Departement de Bacteriologie, Hopital des Enfants, Bordeaux, France

The enzymatic profiles of 97 thermophilic campylobacters were determined by using the micromethod ZYM API-7 which allows a semiquantitative determination of 69 enzymes: 58 arylamidases, 10 esterases and one transpeptidase. The strains studied were those from humans (19), chickens (19), cows (17), sheep (13), pigs (22), dog (one), and reference strains including type strains of **Campylobacter jejuni**, **C. coli** and **C. fetus** subsp. **fetus**. The classical tolerance and biochemical tests were also carried out.

Only 17 enzymes were positive at least once: 11 arylamidases, one transpeptidase and five esterases. Four enzymes were present in all campylobacter strains tested: one arylamidase (L-phenylalanyl-L-proline), three esterases (C_4, C_5, C_6). Five others were very common (64-88%): four arylamidases (L-lysine, glycylglycine, L-alanyl-L-alanyl-L-proline, glycylarginine), one esterase (C_8). Most of the enzymes were present in small amounts. Only three enzymes showed a moderate to strong activity in more than 50% of the strains. The distribution of enzymes was not related to the strain origin nor to the species differentiation (based on hippurate hydrolysis) except for the strong enzymatic activity of the transpeptidase and of the N-benzoyl-L-leucyl arylamidase, which were found respectively in 49% and 43% of **C. jejuni** strains and none in **C. coli**. No relationship has been noted with classical testing. The variability of the profiles obtained allows a differentiation between strains which can be useful for epidemiological purposes. Ten enzymes have been selected for an experimental microgallery CAMPY currently in study.

Sensitivity to irgasan (2,4,4'-trichloro-2'-hydroxydiphenyl ether) in identification of Campylobacter spp.

B. D. Firehammer and M. M. Border

Veterinary Research Laboratory, Montana State University, Bozeman, Montana 59717, USA

Identification of campylobacters is often difficult because of the few differential characteristics available. The problem is becoming more obvious with the isolation of previously undescribed campylobacters from various sources. We have found that differences in sensitivity to the bacteriostatic compound irgasan (2,4,4'-trichloro-2'-hydroxydiphenyl ether) exist between members of the genus. This characteristic may be useful in species differentiation. Minimal inhibitory concentrations of irgasan in broth were determined and two concentrations evaluated by agar dilution:

Organism	No. of isolates	Broth (no. strains growing)					Tryptose blood agar (no. grew/ no. tested)	
		Irgasan conc. (mg/l)					Irgasan conc. (mg/l)	
		2	4	8	16	32	8	128
C. fecalis	14	14	7	0	0	0	12/12	0/15
C. jejuni	19	19	18	0	0	0	6/6	0/26
C. hyointestinalis	8	8	8	3	0	0	4/4	9/9
C. fetus subsp. **venerealis**	11	11	11	10	2	0	17/17	8/20
C. fetus subsp. **fetus**	38	38	38	38	37	23	11/11	21/21

The results indicate that **C. jejuni**, **C. fecalis** and **C. hyointestinalis** are quite susceptible to irgasan but **C. fetus** subsp. **fetus** is resistant; **C. fetus** subsp. **venerealis** is of intermediate susceptibility. The contrast between **C. jejuni** and **C. fetus** subsp. **fetus** is striking. The bacteriostatic effect was reduced on blood agar and all strains tested grew well at the 8 mg/l concentration, although **Proteus** spp. and some other enteric bacteria were inhibited at this level. This would indicate that irgasan may also be useful in selective media for the isolation of campylobacters.

3. Morphological aspects

Flagellar arrangement and comparative morphology of Campylobacter spp. as shown by light and electron microscopy

M. B. Skirrow,* D. R. Purdham† and J. Benjamin*

*Microbiology Department, Worcester Royal Infirmary, Castle Street Branch, Worcester WR1 3AS, and †Department of Medical Microbiology, The Medical School, Edgbaston, Birmingham B15 2TJ, UK

A recently published flagellar staining method [1], which is almost as simple and quick to perform as a Gram stain, was used in conjunction with electron microscopy to study 67 strains of campylobacters and campylobacter-like organisms. Measurements of cell and flagellar wavelength made by light microscopy were, on average, 6% higher than those made by electron microscopy (39 comparisons gave a correlation coefficient (r) of 0.80).

FLAGELLAR CONFIGURATION **Campylobacter jejuni, C. coli, C. laridis,** "CNW" of Sandstedt **et al.** [2], and CLO-1 and CLO-2 (Totten **et al.**, p. 48 in this volume) were predominantly amphitrichate. **C. concisus, C. fecalis, C. hyointestinalis,** aerotolerant group 2 of Neill **et al.** [3], and **C. sputorum** subspp. **sputorum, mucosalis** and **bubulus** were predominantly monotrichate. **C. fetus** subspp. **fetus** and **venerealis** were also mainly monotrichate, but some strains had up to 47% amphitrichate forms. **C. fetus** subsp. **venerealis** (including "var. **intermedius**") was unique in having as many as 10% lophotrichate forms with up to four, or occasionally five, flagella at one or both poles. Lateral flagella at points of cell division were also seen. Occasional cells with two flagella at one pole were seen in **C. fetus** subsp. **fetus, C. fecalis, C. hyointestinalis, C. sputorum** subsp. **bubulus**, and in one strain of **C. laridis.**

CELL AND FLAGELLAR WAVELENGTH The shortest mean cell wavelength values were found in **C. laridis** (940 nm), **C. jejuni** (1020 nm), "CNW" (1120 nm), and **C. coli** (1140 nm); the longest were found in **C. fecalis** (2120 nm), **C. hyointestinalis** (2100 nm), **C. sputorum** subsp. **bubulus** (2090 nm), and **C. fetus** subsp. **venerealis** (2000 nm).

Mean flagellar wavelength was broadly similar in all groups but with a fairly wide range within groups. However, the ratio of cell to flagellar wavelength was surprisingly constant, i.e. a strain with a short cell wavelength (for its group) usually had a short flagellar wavelength, and vice versa. The ratio of cell to flagellar wavelength for most groups was below 0.8, but **C. fecalis, C. sputorum** subsp. **bubulus** and **C. hyointestinalis** were outstanding in having ratios above unity (1.21, 1.15 and 1.03, respectively). Moreover, **C. fecalis** and **C. sputorum** subsp. **bubulus** appeared strikingly similar in that both had unusually long flagella of relatively short wavelength.

REFERENCES

1. H. Kodaka, A. Y. Armfield, G. L. Lombard and V. R. Dowell. Practical procedure for demonstrating bacterial flagella. Journal of Clinical Microbiology, 1982, **16**, 948-952.
2. K. Sandstedt, J. Ursing and M. Walder. Thermotolerant **Campylobacter** with no or weak catalase activity isolated form dogs. Current Microbiology, 1983, **8**, 209-213.
3. S. D. Neill, W. A. Ellis and J. J. O'Brien. Designation of aerotolerant **Campylobacter**-like organisms from porcine and bovine abortions to the genus **Campylobacter**. Research in Veterinary Science, 1979, **27**, 180-186.

Some new structures in the flagellar apparatus of Campylobacter jejuni

A. Curry, **A. J. Fox** and D. M. Jones

Public Health Laboratory, Withington Hospital, Manchester M20 8LR, UK

Campylobacter jejuni is a Gram-negative organism with characteristic comma, S-shaped or sinusoidal profiles. It is flagellated, usually carrying a single flagellar filament at each pole. The outer membrane-like component of the cell wall appears loose fitting except at the poles, where this structure becomes dished and closely associated with the inner, true cytoplasmic membrane. This dish marks the insertion of the flagellar apparatus through the bacterial wall. The hook region of the flagellar apparatus is tapered proximally and is located in the polar concavity. The concave form of this terminal region is maintained by a sub-outer membranous structure. This previously undescribed 110 nm dished structure features a central hole through which the basal apparatus of the flagellum passes and has 11 spoke-like arms radiating from this central hole (the "cartwheel structure"). Partial chemical characterisation of this cartwheel structure has been attempted.

Thin sections of the terminal region of campylobacters show additional structures not found in the rod-shaped Gram-negative bacteria. The inner membrane of the terminal region of campylobacters appears to be a fairly rigid truncated cone 200-300 nm in length. The inner (cytoplasmic) side of the membrane has a 6 nm electron-dense thickening and 10 nm internally to this dense layer is an additional electron-dense cone. Links can be demonstrated between these concentric inner and outer truncated cones. Similar internal structures have been found in some Spirilla and these features may, therefore, be of some taxonomic value.

4. Newly described campylobacters and campylobacter-like organisms

Characterization of human campylobacter-like organisms

C. L. Fennell, P. A. Totten, T. C. Quinn, K. K. Holmes and W. E. Stamm

University of Washington, Seattle, Washington, USA

In studies undertaken to assess possible sexual transmission of **Campylobacter** spp., we isolated three biochemically distinct groups of campylobacter-like organisms (CLO) from homosexual men. In all, CLOs were isolated from 28 of 181 homosexual men with intestinal symptoms versus seven of 77 asymptomatic homosexual men and none of 150 asymptomatic heterosexual men and women. Rectal swabs were inoculated on Brucella agar base medium containing 10% sheep blood, vancomycin, polymixin B, trimethoprim and amphotericin B, which was incubated microaerobically at 37 °C for 7 days. Like catalase-positive **Campylobacter** spp., CLOs were curved Gram-negative rods that did not grow aerobically, were motile, oxidase and catalase positive, and did not utilize glucose. However, strains in each of the three CLO groups differed from previously described **Campylobacter** spp. by at least two growth or biochemical characteristics. CLOs were inhibited by 0.03 mg discs of nalidixic acid and tolerated 1% glycine and 0.04% triphenyltetrazolium chloride, but none grew at 25 °C, hydolyzed hippurate, produced H_2S in TSI, or tolerated 2% NaCl. The three groups were differentiated by nitrate reduction, growth at 42 °C, sensitivity to cephalothin and odor. Thus CLOs cannot be classified within any of the previously described **Campylobacter** spp. Further studies are needed to establish the taxonomic status of CLOs and to clarify their role in gastrointestinal illness.

Genetic characterization of campylobacter-like organisms isolated from homosexual men in Seattle

P. A. Totten, C. L. Fennell, F. Tenover, J. Wezenberg, P. Perine, W. E. Stamm and K. K. Holmes

Departments of Medicine and Epidemiology, University of Washington, the Seattle Public Health Hospital, the Harborview Medical Center and the Veterans Administration Hospital, Seattle, Washington, USA

We have genetically characterized the campylobacter-like organisms (CLOs) isolated from homosexual men in Seattle. These organisms fell into three phenotypically distinct groups, designated CLO-1, CLO-2 and CLO-3, which showed < 10% homology either between groups or with the catalase-positive **Campylobacter** spp. by whole cell DNA homology tests. Eight CLO-1 strains were tested for homology with each other. Seven had > 90% homology when tested under both optimal and stringent conditions, indicating that the DNA of these organisms is highly conserved. One CLO-1 isolate had only 50% DNA homology with the other seven CLO-1 strains, but it could not be differentiated from them biochemically. The two CLO-2 strains tested were also > 90% homologous with each other both under optimal and stringent conditions.

The guanine plus cytosine content of DNA was 37-38 mol% for CLO-1 and CLO-2 strains and 45 mol% for the single CLO-3 isolate. These results place the CLO-1 and CLO-2 strains within, and the CLO-3 strain above, the values obtained for previously described **Campylobacter** spp. (30-38 mol%).

Based on genetic tests, the CLO strains from Seattle can be placed into three species which are genetically distinct from previously characterized catalase-positive **Campylobacter** spp. One of these species (CLO-1) can be further divided genetically into two subspecies.

We have developed a modification of the colony hybridization procedure to differentiate and group new CLO strains rapidly, without having to isolate their DNAs.

Aerotolerant campylobacter: their taxonomic position

S. D. Neill, J. J. O'Brien and W. A. Ellis

Veterinary Research Laboratories, Stoney Road, Stormont, Belfast BT4 3SD, Northern Ireland

In recent years unusual campylobacter-like organisms have been isolated from fetal and placental specimens of different animal species. These isolates have been identified as campylobacters and have DNA base ratios between 29 and 34 mol%. They are different from strains of **Campylobacter fetus**. Their existence has now been recognised in several countries in association with animal reproduction disorders, and hence the potential exists for confusion with **C. fetus** in the diagnosis of "vibrionic abortion" and "venereal vibriosis". Similar strains have also been isolated on a number of occasions from milks of mastitic cows, and mastitis has been reproduced experimentally using one of these isolates.

Sequenced agglomerative hierarchial non-overlapping (SAHN) clustering and ordination methods were used to examine biochemical and physiological data from the aerotolerant strains and authentic campylobacter reference strains. The computer analysis, presented graphically, showed the aerotolerant strains to be a different but heterologous group, clearly different from the existing species and subspecies. The taxonomic novelty of this group has been confirmed using polyacrylamide gel electrophoresis of acid phenol protein extracts and whole cell fatty acid composition data. Strains of this new taxospecies can readily be differentiated from other species by their ability to grow in air, at 15 °C and in the presence of sodium chloride (2%) and carbenicillin (64 mg/l). Attention is drawn to the spectrum-like nature of the genus **Campylobacter** and the drawbacks of employing limited numbers of biochemical and physiological tests are emphasised.

B. ISOLATION AND DETECTION

The detection of Campylobacter jejuni/coli in stools and tissues by an antiserum to a common heat-stable antigen

J. M. Dolby, A. B. Price and P. R. Dunscombe

Clinical Research Centre and Northwick Park Hospital, Watford Road, Harrow, Middlesex HA1 3UJ, UK

An immunofluorescent technique for detecting **Campylobacter jejuni/coli** will be described. It has been tested for its ability to detect campylobacter diagnostically in stools. In a trial of 28 stool specimens from patients with acute diarrhoea, which included cases of proven campylobacter infection, there was agreement between immunofluorescence and culture in 19. Some of the discrepancies can be explained by differences in sensitivity between immunofluorescence and culture; the former could only be interpreted as positive when more than 10^6 organisms per gram of stool were present. In six patients who were culture-negative but immunofluorescence-positive, four had been receiving antibiotics.

The method has now been employed diagnostically on 27 rectal biopsy samples with 70-80% agreement between the fluorescence and culture results. In rectal biopsy samples from 10 bacteriologically proven cases of campylobacter infection, organisms were observed in the lumen of the bowel but not invading the mucosa.

The antigen involved is stable to 100 °C but is not O-specific. It is shared by 50 strains of **C. jejuni**, three strains of **C. coli** and one of **C. laridis** tested. **C. fetus** fluoresces only weakly. Some strains of **Bacteroides fragilis** are positive and cross-reactions have been observed with **Wolinella** spp. Other intestinal pathogens including **Vibrio cholerae** and commensals are negative. An unknown, strongly fluorescent organism has been seen in the stools of two immune-deficient patients with chronic diarrhoea.

The use of an improved fluorescent antibody test and ELISA to detect campylobacters in human stool specimens

D. W. Lambe, Jr and W. F. Campbell

Department of Microbiology, Quillen-Dishner College of Medicine, East Tennessee State University, Johnson City, Tennessee 37614, USA

In 1981, we reported a fluorescent antibody conjugate that stained **Campylobacter jejuni**, but did not react positively with other aerobes or anaerobes. A 1+ fluorescence was positive; this pale fluorescence made the test difficult to read. A new polyvalent FITC conjugate has been developed which reacted positively (3+ to 4+ fluorescence) with 100% of 111 strains of **C. jejuni** and with 100% of 36 strains of **C. coli**. **C. fetus**, **C. intestinalis**, other aerobes and anaerobes were negative. Organisms in human stool samples from patients infected with **C. jejuni** also gave positive fluorescence.

A solid-phase enzyme-linked immunosorbent assay (ELISA) was developed to identify **C. jejuni**. In the assay, hyperimmune mouse and rabbit anti-**C. jejuni** sera exhibited titers of nearly 1:1,000,000 and 1:100,000 respectively. Using peroxidase-conjugated goat anti-rabbit immunoglobulin (or rabbit anti-mouse immunoglobulin) and OPD, the assay detected 5-20 ng of bacterial protein from pure cultures of **C. jejuni**. When whole bacteria were examined, antisera were unable to distinguish strains of **C. jejuni** from those of **C. coli**. However, ELISA differentiated **C. jejuni** from **C. coli** if SDS-treated outer membranes (OM) were used in the assay. Rabbits were immunized with SDS-treated OM preparations derived from **C. jejuni** or **C. coli**. The anti-**C. jejuni** OM serum reacted specifically with **C. jejuni** whole bacteria. The ELISA detected **C. jejuni** when these strains were inoculated into fresh, normal stool specimens. There was an inhibitory factor in stools more than 1 day old.

Use of a DNA probe to detect Campylobacter jejuni in fecal specimens

L. S. Tompkins, P. Mickelsen and J. McClure

Departments of Microbiology and Immunology and Laboratory Medicine, University of Washington School of Medicine, Seattle, Washington 98195, USA

We have developed a rapid method to detect **Campylobacter jejuni** in clinical materials directly by colony hybridization employing a specific DNA probe. Stool samples are spotted on to nitrocellulose filters which are hybridized directly without allowing colonies to develop. A preliminary study using a probe consisting of **C. jejuni** chromosomal fragments radiolabeled by nick translation showed that the probe reacted with **C. jejuni** but not with other **Campylobacter** species, other bacterial pathogens, or normal fecal flora. This probe was then applied to nitrocellulose filters which had been spotted with 299 diarrheal stool samples, 18 of which were culture positive. The probe detected 10 of these, giving a sensitivity of 44% and a positive predictive value of 34%. Fifteen of 281 culture negative samples were probe positive (specificity 94%; negative predictive value 96%). None of the samples containing salmonellas, shigellas or yersinias were probe positive. The probe was able to detect no fewer than 1×10^7 organisms per milliliter of feces.

In order to enhance the sensitivity of the method we constructed a second probe consisting of eight unique chromosomal fragments ranging in size from 7–11 kb which were cloned into pBR322. After digestion of the clones with Hind III and Bam H1, the fragments were subjected to electrophoresis, eluted on to DEAE cellulose paper, purified and nick translated. The effect of dextran sulfate on enhancing sensitivity was also examined. The effect of treatment to deproteinize fecal samples with dithiothreotol was examined and showed no effect on sensitivity. The addition of dextran sulfate to the hybridization reaction enhanced sensitivity 10-fold so that as few as 1×10^7–2×10^7 **C. jejuni** per milliliter of stool could be detected. Incubation of **C. jejuni** seeded into TSY broth and incubated on filters over Campy agar enhanced sensitivity of detection, whereas **C. jejuni** suspended in feces failed to replicate as well, suggesting the presence of inhibitors in fecal material. There was no advantage in using the pooled cloned fragment probes over the chromosomal probe, in that both probes could detect no less than 2×10^6 organisms per milliliter of stool. Fecal material tends to reduce sensitivity and specificity of hybridization compared with broth. Although the chromosomal probe applied to stool samples directly spotted onto filters gave a low sensitivity, the high specificity of the probe warrants further efforts to reduce the effect of substances in the stool which contribute to false positivity and interfere with DNA hybridization.

Sub-lethal injury and campylobacters

T. J. Humphrey and J. G. Cruickshank

Public Health Laboratory, Church Lane, Heavitree, Exeter, Devon EX2 5AD, UK

While campylobacters are readily isolated from animal faeces, their detection in chilled, refrigerated or frozen foods known to be faecally contaminated is more difficult. Low temperatures can cause sub-lethal injury in enterobacteria and may amongst other things render the organisms more sensitive to antibiotics. The effect of such temperatures on the sensitivity of campylobacters to some antibiotics used in selective isolation media was studied.

When log phase cultures of **Campylobacter jejuni** biotype 1 were stored at +4 °C or −20 °C, 75% and 94% of the population were killed in 4 h respectively. The survivors, incubated on blood agar at 43 °C for 48 h, produced atypical colonies. The ability to grow normally with recognisable colonial form was recovered after 4 h in broth at 43 °C. Those organisms surviving low temperature storage for 24 h were more sensitive to rifampicin at 42 °C and to polymyxin at 37 °C, resulting in lower counts on blood agar in which these antibiotics were incorporated.

When cells, thawed after 24 h at -20 °C, were incubated in broth at 43 °C there was an initial decrease in the number of viable cells. The magnitude of the fall varied from serotype to serotype. With Penner serotype 2 strains the death rate and subsequent growth was unaffected by the presence of rifampicin or polymixin. Conversely, serotype 4 strains recovered more quickly in the presence of polymyxin, although cells in the control broths with no antibiotics or in broths containing rifampicin declined to undetectable levels within 6 h!

A blood-free selective medium for the isolation of campylobacters

F. J. Bolton, D. N. Hutchinson and D. C. Coates

Public Health Laboratory, Royal Infirmary, Meadow Street, Preston PR1 6PS, UK

A blood-free selective agar has been developed which contains Nutrient Broth No. 2 (Oxoid) 25 g/l, New Zealand agar (Davies) 12 g/l, casein hydrolysates (Oxoid) 3 g/l, Bacteriological Charcoal (Oxoid) 4 g/l, ferrous sulphate 0.25 g/l, sodium pyruvate 0.25 g/l, sodium deoxycholate (BDH) 1 g/l and cephazolin (Eli Lilly) 10,000 mg/l (CCD agar). Screening tests on 50 possible selective agents indicated that sodium deoxycholate and cephazolin were the most suitable for inclusion in the blood-free agar. Selective supplements described by other workers may not be compatible with the charcoal basal medium.

The CCD agar was compared with the Preston medium for isolation of **Campylobacter jejuni** from approx. 1000 human faecal specimens. Isolation rates on both media were similar, and although CCD agar was less selective this did not interfere with the isolation of campylobacters from positive specimens. Temperature studies at 37 °C and 42 °C confirmed that incubation of direct plates at 42 °C for 48 h was necessary for maximum isolation of **C. jejuni**.

A blood-free selective enrichment broth was also prepared which has a similar formulation except for the omission of agar and the addition of sodium metabisulphite 0.25 g/l. This enrichment broth was compared with the modified Preston enrichment broth for the isolation of campylobacters from human faeces and environmental samples. These studies confirmed the value of enrichment culture and indicated that the use of the blood-free enrichment medium and the modified Preston enrichment broth in conjunction give optimum yields.

Optimal isolation of Campylobacter jejuni in developing countries in relation to cost and efficiency

H. Goossens, M. De Boeck, A. Daems and J. P. Butzler

WHO Collaborating Centre for **Campylobacter jejuni** and Department of Microbiology, St Pierre University Hospital, Hoogstraat 322, 1000 Brussels, Belgium

Campylobacter jejuni can now be isolated from faecal specimens with low costs in modestly equipped laboratories, which is extremely important in developing countries where **Campylobacter** is becoming a major enteropathogen. We are able to prove that, even after advanced economy, isolation techniques can still be reliable. This premise is based on studies which have been carried out in our laboratory during the last two years.

MEDIA We developed a new selective medium, Butzler's Medium Virion (BMV), since Skirrow medium, Butzler's Medium Oxoid (BMO) and Campy-BAP are not sufficiently inhibitory on pseudomonas and some Enterobacteriaceae. We have found that BMV, compared with BMO, allows easier reading of plates and better recognition of campylobacters. This new selective medium has now been commercialised.

INCUBATION Incubation in a candle jar or a plastic bag gives extremely favourable results, even without adding FBP supplement to the medium. With BMV, plates can be incubated at 37 °C, since there is no difference in isolation of **C. jejuni** and in the growth of competing faecal flora compared with incubation at 42 °C.

EXAMINATION OF PLATES Some 99.2% of **C. jejuni** can be found in stools within 2 days of incubation at 37 °C if the agar concentration in BMV is reduced to 10.5 g/l. Therefore, plates need no longer be incubated at 42 °C or for more than 2 days.

IDENTIFICATION The characteristic morphology can be observed with a Vago stain (a colouration with eosin 2% and crystal violet), which is usually sufficient for identification.

STORAGE AND TRANSPORT A simple procedure was shown to be successful: a thioglycollate medium, inoculated with campylobacters, is dispensed in small amounts into upright tubes, which are then covered with paraffin wax. The tubes are closed with a lid which is screwed down.

Thus, the isolation, identification, storage and transport of **C. jejuni** from faecal specimens has become a simple and cheap, yet reliable procedure.

Evaluation of four different methods for the isolation of thermophilic campylobacter species from stool specimens

H. W. Van Landuyt, N. I. Mestdagh and **J. M. Fossepre**

A.Z. St Jan, Department of Microbiology, Ruddershovelaan 10, B-8000 Brugge, Belgium

During a 7 month period, 1407 unselected stool specimens submitted to the clinical laboratory were simultaneously cultured by four different methods. Each sample was plated on to Butzler's campylobacter selective agar and Blaser's campylobacter selective agar. Incubation took place at 42 °C for 48 h both in a candle jar and in a polyethylene bag for Butzler's medium, but only in a candle jar for Blaser's medium. The bag was filled by exhaling into it and sealing with a rubber band. The effect of enrichment was studied by inoculating a thioglycollate medium USP (Oxoid CM173) supplemented with Skirrow's campylobacter selective supplement (Oxoid SR69) and 0.16% agar (Difco 0140). The thioglycollate broth was left overnight in a refrigerator, subcultured on to Butzler's medium and incubated at 42 °C for 48 h in a candle jar.

A total of 51 (3.6%) campylobacter isolates was obtained. Of these isolates 44 (86.3%) were identified as **C. jejuni** and seven (13.7%) were identified as **C. coli**. Butzler's medium incubated in a candle jar accounted for 46 (90.2%) of the 51 isolates, whereas 40 strains (78.4%) were isolated with the same medium incubated in the polyethylene bag. Thirty-two strains (62.7%) were isolated on Blaser's medium (candle jar) and only 21 isolates (41.2%) were obtained after thioglycollate enrichment. No distinctive difference between the isolation of **C. jejuni** and **C. coli** could be found with respect to the different media employed.

From this study it can be concluded that Butzler's medium incubated at 42 °C in a candle jar for 48 h gives a higher isolation rate than either Blaser's medium under similar conditions or Butzler's medium incubated in a polyethylene bag. Furthermore, enrichment in the thioglycollate broth as a single isolation method for thermophilic campylobacters has to be discouraged.

The use of membrane filters applied directly to the surface of agar plates for the isolation of Campylobacter jejuni from faeces

T. W. Steele and S. N. McDermott

Institute of Medical and Veterinary Science, Box 14, Rundle Street PO, Adelaide, South Australia 5000, Australia

Membrane filtration has been used successfully to isolate campylobacters from faeces in the past. This has required special apparatus and has frequently been combined with selective antibiotic media when used as a routine isolation method. For two years we have used 450 nm Gelman filters applied directly to the surface of dried 7% sheep blood agar plates for the routine isolation of campylobacters in our laboratory in Adelaide, South Australia. A saline suspension of faeces is prepared and 10 drops are placed on the filter with care being taken to prevent flow over the edge of the membrane. The filter is removed after 30 min, by which time the fluid has passed through to the agar medium. The plates are incubated in microaerobic conditions at 43 °C for 3 days.

We examined 1000 faecal specimens using this technique in parallel with our selective antibiotic medium. Of 56 isolates of campylobacter, 50 were detected by filter and 45 by antibiotic medium. The sensitivity was 89% and 80% respectively. This simple filter method which uses unselective readily available laboratory media is as effective as currently available methods. It permits the isolation of antibiotic sensitive strains of **Campylobacter jejuni**. In addition it aids the isolation of other thermophilic campylobacters from patients with diarrhoea. It will provide an opportunity for expansion of our knowledge of the ecology and pathogenic role of these bacteria.

Enrichment media for Campylobacter jejuni: a systematic investigation

V. D. Bokkenheuser

Department of Microbiology, St Luke's-Roosevelt Hospital Center, Amsterdam Avenue at 114th Street, New York, New York 10025, USA

In preliminary experiments it was shown that thioglycollate broth required a median of 15 colony-forming units (c.f.u.) and Mueller-Hinton broth more than 200 c.f.u. of stock strains of **Campylobacter jejuni** for growth. Addition of whole horse or sheep blood increased the sensitivity but best results were obtained with 5% lysed sheep blood in thioglycollate broth (TLS). TLS supplemented with Blaser's antibiotic mixture required a median of 15 c.f.u. for growth. TLS supplemented with Butzler's antibiotic mixture required a median of 25 c.f.u. and three strains failed to grow with an inoculum of 200 c.f.u. The enhanced inhibition of Butzler's antibiotic mixture was abolished by addition of 0.1% lauryl sulfate. Since TLS with Butzler's antibiotic mixture suppressed growth of non-campylobacter organisms better than TLS with Blaser's mixture, the former was adopted for further studies with wild strains of **C. jejuni**. Thus organisms were obtained by selective filtration (650 nm) of diluted cecal content from newly slaughtered chickens. The TLS-Butzler-lauryl sulfate enrichment broth required an inoculum of 1 c.f.u. of wild strains of **C. jejuni**, as did Blaser's selective agar and chocolate agar. The sensitivity of the enrichment medium could be increased by increasing the size of the inoculum; for example, 50 ml of enrichment broth seeded with a 5 ml sample was 50 times more sensitive than chocolate agar seeded with 0.1 ml of the same suspension of wild strains of **C. jejuni**. Double strength enrichment broth was less sensitive to **C. jejuni** than single strength enrichment broth.

Enrichment medium for the isolation of Campylobacter jejuni from stools – an update on laboratory findings

F. T. H. Chan and A. M. R. Mackenzie

Department of Laboratory Medicine, Children's Hospital of Eastern Ontario, 401 Smyth Road, Ottawa, Ontario K1H 8L1, Canada

An enrichment medium consisting of semi-solid motility test medium, 7% lysed horse blood, vancomycin 10 mg/l, polymyxin B 5 mg/l and trimethoprim 5 mg/l was used, in addition to primary plating, to isolate **Campylobacter jejuni** from stools. After overnight incubation the enrichment medium was subcultured to selective plates which were then incubated in jars at 42 °C in an atmosphere of 5% O_2, 10% CO_2 and 85% N_2.

Over a 5 year period (1978–82), 266 faecal specimens from 218 patients were positive to campylobacters. The enrichment medium yielded all 266 isolates, whereas primary plating produced only 243 positives, indicating that 23 isolates (8.6%) would have been missed if the enrichment technique was not used. These 23 enrichment isolates were from 21 patients, 19 of whom had symptoms. Of the remaining two patients, one was a known case diagnosed 2 months previously and the other was asymptomatic. Twelve of these 21 patients were within 3 days of onset of symptoms, whereas eight symptomatic patients had a history ranging from 1 week to 7 months. Six patients were treated with antibiotics (ampicillin, amoxycillin or erythromycin) before specimen collection.

This study demonstrates the advantage of using enrichment culture for campylobacters. Enrichment methods may be necessary to isolate **C. jejuni** in some cases and might be particularly useful for examination of contacts and follow-up of patients.

Some recent advances in the diagnosis of Campylobacter fetus subsp. venerealis infection in cattle

K. P. Lander,* K. P. W. Gill* and P. I. Hewson†

*Ministry of Agriculture, Fisheries and Food, Central Veterinary Laboratory, New Haw, Weybridge, UK, and †Ministry of Agriculture, Fisheries and Food, Animal Health Office, Castle House, Newport Road, Stafford, UK

The laboratory diagnosis of venereal **Campylobacter fetus** infections in cattle ("bovine venereal vibriosis") presents many problems. Even in laboratories with considerable experience of such diagnoses, results are often disappointing. The main problems include (i) poor standards of samples; (ii) difficulties in maintaining the viability of the organisms in transit; (iii) the need to use techniques unfamiliar to routine diagnostic laboratories and (iv) shortcomings in laboratory diagnostic methods.

Work has been aimed at improving current laboratory tests and developing techniques which can readily be adopted by field or laboratory workers even if they lack experience in the diagnosis of bovine venereal vibriosis. Possible improvements have been made in the following areas:

(1) **Collection of samples** (a) Preputial exudate in bulls - if a lavage technique is used, the need to massage the prepuce and penis vigorously cannot be overemphasised. (b) Cervicovaginal mucus in cows - a new lavage technique is simple to use, very effective, safe for the collector and for the cow and gives a sample which is easy to process [1].

(2) **Culture** (a) A modified Skirrow's agar is a very effective medium for isolating **C. fetus**. (b) Culture of vaginal mucus from cows is a valuable aid to diagnosis. (c) A transport and enrichment medium greatly facilitates culture from bulls and cows.

(3) **Detection of antibodies in mucus** An enzyme-linked immunosorbent assay (ELISA) for antibodies in cervicovaginal mucus is more sensitive and detects antibodies earlier than the commonly used mucus agglutination test. (See abstract on p. 74.)

REFERENCE

1. K. P. Lander. New techniques for collection of vaginal mucus from cattle. Veterinary Research, 1983, **112**, 570.

Session III

ANTIGENS AND SERODIAGNOSIS

Report on the Session

ANTIGENS

The techniques of sodium dodecyl sulphate polyacrylamide gel electrophoresis, immunoblotting, radioimmunoprecipitation, radiolabelling and the preparation of monoclonal antibodies against surface antigens were among the techniques used by contributors to examine the complexity of the surface antigens of **Campylobacter jejuni** and the reactivity of some of the determinants to antisera and to human convalescent sera. The presence of many major and minor outer membrane and flagellar proteins was demonstrated on the gels that were shown. There was agreement on the presence of an outer membrane component of approximately 30,000 daltons, removable by glycine extraction, antigenic and cross-reactive with different sera. Another band of approximately 44,000 daltons was constantly present and represented the majority of the protein present in the preparations. This protein was also cross-reactive and antibody to it was demonstrated in human convalescent sera. Antibody to this protein was also shown to be present in samples of cord blood, human breast milk and human bile. Bands associated with the flagellar apparatus were of high molecular weight, 62,000-66,000 daltons, and there were also further associated bands in the 87,000-90,000 dalton range. Using monoclonal antibodies (Logan and Trust, p. 69; Newell, p. 70) at least four determinants were distinguishable as associated with the flagellar apparatus, some of the structural complexities of which had been demonstrated by electron microscopy (Curry **et al.**, p. 46). It seemed possible that one flagellar determinant (in the 92,500 dalton band) might have serotype specificity, but this was not definitely established for a range of serotypes. Such a high molecular weight antigen would be a candidate for involvement in the slide agglutination serotyping system (Lior). If the flagella are involved in some way in the pathogenesis of **C. jejuni** enteritis (and there is some evidence that aflagellate strains are of reduced virulence), a specific flagellar antigen may, amongst others, confer serotype-specific immunity. The high molecular weight protein (97,000 daltons) that was shown to be an anti-phagocyte factor for **C. fetus** by McCoy was not demonstrated in any of the extracts of **C. jejuni**.

Surface antigens in the low molecular weight bands (12,000-21,000 daltons) were demonstrated to be lipopolysaccharide and it was further shown that these conferred antigenic specificity for the strains. By extracting a range of antigens from the gels and using the extracts to sensitise red cells, it was shown that only the lipopolysaccharide antigens are involved in serotyping by passive haemagglutination and confirmed for several serotypes that it is the lipopolysaccharide that confers serotype specificity in this system. Extracted lipopolysaccharide was shown to neutralise most of the homologous bactericidal activity of human convalescent serum, so it is possible that lipopolysaccharide is an antigen involved in the development of serotype-specific immunity.

Monoclonal antibodies were applied to the analysis of some of the cell surface determinants, not only flagellar antigens as previously mentioned, but clones reactive to a variety of other surface antigens were also described. Among these were those that reacted specifically by passive haemagglutination (anti-LPS) and others that reacted specifically by slide agglutination, thus establishing the possiblity of using monoclonal antibodies in definitive typing systems.

THE DETECTION OF ANTIBODIES TO CAMPYLOBACTERS

Application of serological techniques has become well established since the last Workshop. The techniques used by the contributors include agglutination, complement fixation, ELISA, bactericidal assay and radioimmunoassay. Antigens of broad reactivity (sonicates, glycine extracts), both laboratory-produced and commercially available, were found to be useful for the detection of infection; the complement fixation test and ELISA being generally the most useful techniques. However, the variability of the antibody response indicates that the use of more than one technique is preferable in order to detect the maximum number of antibody responses. Homotypic strains were required for the detection of serotype-specific antibody. Contributors assessed their systems by comparing sera from isolate-positive cases with controls (blood donors, antenatal clinic sera, healthy children). It was useful to establish the prevalence of antibody titres in communities both as controls and for studying the effect of dietary differences between communities. There were some estimates of the duration of the antibody response after infection and agreement that about 7-8 months after a single infection antibodies are no longer detectable by the techniques used. It was found when studying outbreaks that a small proportion of those infected did not produce antibody. It was also shown that in some cirumstances between 20 and 50% of those infected with **C. jejuni** may not develop systems.

The radioimmunoassay used by Mascart-Lemone **et al.** (see p. 71) demonstrated that polymeric IgA could frequently be detected in convalescent sera. The future elucidation of the clinical relevance and specificities of this response should yield some interesting information. The ELISA technique was described in a very simple, cheap and storable form by Lior and Lacroix (see p. 72), the test being carried out on nitrocellulose paper. Although no extensive applications were quoted, this test appears to be sensitive for the detection of IgG and IgM and may prove useful for field studies. In the veterinary field the conventional ELISA technique was found to be both sensitive and useful for detecting antibody to **C. fetus** in bovine vaginal mucus (Gill **et al.**, p. 74).

D. M. Jones

Public Health Laboratory,
Manchester, UK

J. R. Davies

Public Health Laboratory Service,
London, UK

Abstracts of Papers Presented

A. ANTIGENS

1. Surface antigens

Molecular identification of the surface antigens of Campylobacter jejuni

S. M. Logan and **T. J. Trust**

Department of Biochemistry and Microbiology, University of Victoria, Victoria, British Columbia V8W 2Y2, Canada

Immunoblotting was used to identify surface antigens of **Campylobacter jejuni**. Polyclonal antiserum was raised in rabbits to formalised cells of a typical human faecal isolate, **C. jejuni** VC74. Surface components were separated by sodium dodecyl sulphate-polyacrylamide gel electrophoresis. Fractions analysed included whole cell lysates, sarcosinate-extracted outer membranes (OM), released OM blebs (fragments), isolated flagella, 0.2 M glycine HCl (pH 2.2) extract, saline extract and material released by osmotic shocking. The ability of the antisera to recognise corresponding antigens on other strains of thermophilic campylobacters and **C. fetus** was determined.

The results demonstrated that antigenic specificity could be conferred by the lipopolysaccharide. Protein antigens were also identified. Both the major OM protein and flagella were immunogenic, but did not confer either strain or species serospecificity on the strains tested. By contrast, an outer membrane protein of molecular weight 92,500 daltons did confer strain-dependent serospecificity in the case of **C. jejuni** VC74.

Another major antigen on thermophilic campylobacter cells was a surface protein of approximate molecular weight 31,000 daltons. This common antigen was preferentially removed by glycine extraction, but was not detectable in OM prepared by sarcosinate extraction.

Antigenic characterisation of outer membrane proteins of Campylobacter jejuni

S. D. Mills, W. C. Bradbury and J. L. Penner

Department of Microbiology, 120 College Street, University of Toronto, Toronto, Ontario M5S 1A1, Canada

The outer membrane (OM) proteins of **Campylobacter jejuni** were studied for their possible involvement during human infection. OM proteins prepared by the EDTA-lysozyme and sarkosyl-insoluble extraction methods were compared by SDS-PAGE and Coomassie brilliant blue (CBB) staining. Two major protein bands of 44,000 and 61,000 daltons and six to 10 minor bands ranging from 14,000 to 92,500 daltons were observed using either technique. SDS-PAGE analysis of released fragments isolated by differential centrifugation revealed a similar protein profile to the OM, except that there was an increased number of bands in the 50,000-70,000 dalton range. Electron microscopy showed that released fragments consisted of pleomorphic vesicles and flagella.

The antigenic nature of the proteins prepared from **C. jejuni** strains isolated during an infection was determined using sera collected before and after infection. These sera were incubated with proteins transferred to nitrocellulose (Western blot) and the antibody-protein complexes were detected with ^{125}I-staphylococcal protein A (immuno-autoradiography). A number of proteins, including the 61,000 and 45,000 dalton major OM proteins, were antigenic and there were changes in the immune blot profiles during the course of infection.

Characterisation of the antigens of Campylobacter jejuni associated with (a) serotyping by haemagglutination and (b) serum bactericidal activity

J. Eldridge, **A. J. Fox** and D. M. Jones

Public Health Laboratory, Withington Hospital, Manchester M20 8LR, UK

(a) SEROTYPING BY HAEMAGGLUTINATION

The haemagglutination system for serotyping **Campylobacter jejuni/coli** depends on heat-stable soluble antigens. We have attempted to characterise the antigens involved in this typing system. Outer membrane components were prepared from whole cells by sodium lauryl sarcosinate extraction for Penner serotypes 1-5. These preparations were run on sodium deodecyl sulphate-polyacrylamide gels and a number of protein/glycoprotein bands were resolved. The gels were cut into 5 mm segments, eluted and then the eluates were dialysed and used to sensitise red cells for the haemagglutination reaction. Haemagglutinating activity was located only in bands within the molecular weight range 10,000-25,000 daltons.

Boiled culture supernatant fluids from the same five serotypes, as prepared for serotyping, were similarly examined by SDS-PAGE. Two major components were present, one of which was located in the 10,000-25,000 dalton range. These two bands were separately eluted and the haemagglutinating activity was present only in the 10,000-25,000 dalton bands.

Lipopolysaccharide from each of the strains was prepared by phenol-water extraction. These were then examined by SDS-PAGE and they each gave a single band within the 10,000-25,000 dalton range, staining with PAS-Schiff. When the bands were eluted serotype-specific haemagglutinating activity was present in the eluate. Thus the active haemagglutinating principle was established.

The same preparations were used in a haemagglutination/inhibition test and these further confirmed that the serotyping reaction depended solely on lipopolysaccharide in the five serotypes examined. Using these techniques the relationships between cross-reacting serotypes 4, 13, 16 and 50 have been investigated.

(b) SERUM BACTERICIDAL ACTIVITY

In the serological response to **C. jejuni** infection, bactericidal antibodies are produced by most, but not all, those infected. What part this antibody has in immunity is still obscure. The antibody is bactericidal to strains of the infecting serotype but not to other serotypes. Using hyperimmune sera this reaction can be used for serotyping strains of **C. jejuni**, and the specificity of the reaction closely resembles that of passive haemagglutination where the cells are sensitised by soluble heat-stable antigen (lipopolysaccharide). We therefore investigated the possibility that lipopolysaccharide (LPS) is also the target antigen for bactericidal antibody.

Supernatants from heated cell suspensions (as for serotyping by haemagglutination) and LPS prepared by phenol-water extraction have been examined to see if they have the ability to neutralise the bactericidal antibody in both rabbit and human sera.

Homologous LPS neutralises the bactericidal activity which appears to be unaffected by heterologous LPS. We have confirmed that LPS is a surface antigen exposed on the whole bacterial cell and available to antibody by electron microscopic studies using a protein A-gold method. The possibility that there are also additional target antigens for bactericidal antibody is being explored.

Campylobacter jejuni outer membrane proteins are antigenic for humans

M. J. Blaser, J. A. Hopkins and M. L. Vasil

Infectious Disease Section, VA Medical Center, and Division of Infectious Diseases, University of Colorado School of Medicine, Denver, Colorado, USA

We have prepared outer membrane-enriched fractions of **Campylobacter jejuni** cells using sarcosyl digestion of crude membrane, or by harvesting membrane vesicles (blebs). Outer membrane protein (OMP) profiles of the bleb and sarcosyl preparation for each strain were similar. All **C. jejuni** strains have a major OMP (mOMP), representing more than 90% of protein present, that migrates between 41,000 and 44,000 daltons. Great variation in minor band profiles was present.

In order to assess whether any of the OMPs were antigenic, we studied serum from rabbits hyperimmunized with **C. jejuni** cells, from humans convalescent after **C. jejuni** infection, and from appropriate controls. Using SDS-solubilized fractions of extrinsically ^{125}I-radiolabelled **C. jejuni** cells we performed a radioimmunoprecipitation (RIP) procedure with the test serum. In this assay the mOMP was the major antigen for both homologously and heterologously immunized rabbits. Minor bands at 30,000, 50,000 and 59,000 daltons were also antigenic. The mOMP was antigenic for 10 sera from naturally infected humans but minimally so for control sera. We tested the same sera in a Western blot procedure using protein A-containing **Staphylococcus aureus** or specific anti-IgA, anti-IgG or anti-IgM conjugates. Both homologous and heterologous rabbit serum, but not control serum, recognized a large number of membrane proteins migrating between 15,000 and 91,000 daltons, but the most antigenic site was the mOMP. Infected humans showed IgA, IgG and IgM antibody responses to the mOMP and several minor bands that were significantly greater than that of controls.

Our data suggest that there is antigenic similarity between mOMPs of different **C. jejuni** strains and that since **C. jejuni** mOMP is universally recognized by infected animals and humans it has potential as a vaccine candidate.

The surface protein antigens including flagella of Campylobacter jejuni

D. G. Newell

Public Health Laboratory, Southampton General Hospital, Southampton, UK

The outer membrane proteins of **Campylobacter jejuni/coli** have been identified by ^{125}I-surface labelling. The major ^{125}I-labelled proteins included a major outer membrane protein of variable molecular weight (43,000-46,000 daltons) and several constant proteins (27,000, 35,000, 64,000 and 72,000 daltons). Outer membranes have been isolated by sucrose density gradient centrifugation of spheroplasts and by sarkosyl extraction. The two preparations are comparable but the former contains more proteins. Several proteins, especially the 27,000 and 72,000 dalton proteins were surface ^{125}I-labelled but were not recovered in the isolated outer membranes. One protein in the outer membranes appears to have a molecular weight of 35,000 daltons in **C. jejuni** strains and 41,000 daltons in **C. coli** strains. The molecular weight (62,000 daltons) of flagella was determined using isolated flagella and confirmed with an aflagellate variant. A protein of molecular weight 84,000 daltons is probably hook protein as it is a minor contaminant of flagella and is also absent in the aflagellate variant.

Some of the surface antigens have been identified by radioimmunoprecipitation and immunoblotting. Because flagella are not ^{125}I-labelled using the iodogen or lactoperoxidase iodination techniques a method has been established to ^{125}I-label flagella using methyl [3,5,-^{125}I]iodohydroxybenzimidate. Both the major outer membrane protein and flagella are major antigens detected by sera from immunised rabbits. Moreover homologous and heterologous human convalescent sera immunoprecipitate significantly more ^{125}I-labelled major outer membrane protein and flagella than control sera. The 27,000 dalton protein was also precipitated by some human sera.

Monoclonal antibodies directed against flagella suggest that there are at least four antigenic determinants on flagella but that only one is common to all **C. jejuni** strains.

Our studies indicate that both flagella and the major outer membrane protein are immunogenic during naturally acquired human infections and that some of the antibodies produced during these infections are cross-reacting.

Biochemical and immunological analysis of the antigenic material removed by heat from Campylobacter jejuni

G. E. Buck, J. S. Smith and K. A. Parshall

Department of Pathology, University of Texas Medical Branch, Galveston, Texas 77550, USA

The material removed from **Campylobacter jejuni** by boiling whole cells in saline was analyzed to investigate its antigenic and biochemical composition. The antigen preparation was prepared by growing the organism on Columbia Blood Agar Base for 24 h at 37 °C, then suspending the cells in 0.15 M saline and boiling for 1 h. The bacteria were removed by centrifugation and filtration.

Extracts prepared in this manner contained three antigenic components, as determined by two-dimensional immunodiffusion and crossed immunoelectrophoresis. Biochemical analysis showed that the extract contained 3.04 mg/l of protein and 2.57 mg/l of carbohydrate per milligram (wet weight) of cells. Further extraction with chloroform-methanol produced an average of 0.56 mg/l of material, suggesting the presence of lipid as well.

Electrophoresis on polyacrylamide gel revealed five to seven bands in gels without sodium dodecyl sulfate (SDS), and at least 10 bands in gels with SDS. The extract was positive when tested by the limulus lysate assay, suggesting the presence of lipopolysaccharide O antigen. The results suggest that this antigen complex is the outer membrane of the cell, although additional work will be required to prove this conclusively.

Characteristics of the thermostable antigens of Campylobacter jejuni

M. A. Preston, J. L. Penner and W. C. Bradbury

Department of Microbiology, University of Toronto, Toronto, Ontario M5G 1L5, Canada

Isolates of **Campylobacter jejuni** can be differentiated on the basis of 42 antigens that are resistant to heat, and a serotyping scheme based on the specificities of these antigens is under development. Antigenic material was obtained from several serotype reference strains using the hot phenol-water technique for extracting lipopolysaccharides (LPS). These extracts were used to sensitise sheep erythrocytes for passive haemagglutination (PHA) titrations of serotyping antisera.

The immunological specificities of these extracts were found to be indistinguishable from the specificities of the antigens extracted from the same strains by heating saline suspensions of bacteria. In addition, phenol-water extracts were analysed by fractionating their components by sodium dodecyl sulphate polyacrylamide gel eletrophoresis (SDS-PAGE) and visualising them with a silver stain modified for LPS. Electrophoresis material from different strains had profiles characteristic of both smooth (O+) and rough (O-) LPS antigens. These procedures were used to investigate the LPS structure of strains exhibiting cross-reactivity in PHA titrations.

The results indicated that the specificities of the thermostable antigens used as markers in a serotyping scheme were due to the somatic (O) LPS antigens characteristic of Gram-negative bacteria.

Immunological and biochemical characterization of Campylobacter jejuni whole cell and subcellar fractions

J. P. Burans, S. D. Stewart and A. L. Bourgeois

Naval Medical Research Institute, Bethesda, Maryland, USA, and Naval Medical Research Unit Three, Cairo, Egypt

Protein and LPS profiles of whole cell (WC) preparations of campylobacter isolates were obtained by SDS-PAGE. Whereas each isolate had a unique protein profile, significant relatedness was demonstrated. Two prominent protein bands (45,000 and 61,000 daltons) were present in all **C. jejuni** and **C. coli** isolates. Immunodetection of Western blot (WB) of WC preparations with rabbit hyperimmune serum to **C. jejuni** (ATCC 29428) demonstrated the immunogenicity of the proteins. Immunodetection of WB of **C. jejuni** WC preparations with convalescent sera from infected rabbits and humans gave similar results. Correlation was observed between the intensity of the 61,000 dalton immunodetected band and reactivity of hyperimmune serum with WC preparations in ELISA. One **C. fetus** isolate examined had a unique protein profile and was the least reactive isolate on the immunodetected WB ELISA.

LPS profiles of **C. jejuni** and **C. coli** were obtained using a modified silver stain unreactive to protein. LPS bands of varying size and intensity were detected only in the 14,000-21,000 dalton gel regions. These profiles suggested the presence of short chain LPS without significant O-side chain branching. The **C. fetus** isolate had a unique LPS profile: one LPS complex was observed in the 14,000-21,000 dalton gel region as well as a two-band complex in the 21,000-30,000 dalton gel region suggestive of the presence of O-side chains of intermediate length. WC preparations and subcellular fractions, including purified membrane isolated without detergents, were studied by SDS-PAGE and two-dimensional PAGE. Increased complexity of protein profiles was observed following separation based upon isoelectric point and molecular weight.

2. Monoclonal antibodies

Serotyping and antigenic analysis of campylobacters with monoclonal antibodies

T. U. Kosunen, B. Bang and M. Hurme

Department of Bacteriology and Immunology, University of Helsinki, Haartmaninkatu 3, 00290 Helsinki 29, Finland

Enzyme immunoassay with live bacteria as antigen was used to screen for monoclonal antibodies against campylobacters obtained by fusion of mouse myeloma cells with spleen cells from mice immunised with formalin-treated bacteria. Of the 29 antibodies (ascites) obtained against **Campylobacter jejuni** strain 143483, 13 reacted with the immunogen in one or more of the following tests: slide agglutination of live bacteria, tube agglutination of boiled bacteria, passive haemagglutination (PHA) with saline extracts and a purified polysaccharide preparation as the antigen, and enzyme immunoassay with an acid glycine extract as the antigen.

The acid extract seems to contain a common antigen for campylobacters, since the clone that gave the strongest reaction with it, reacted also with all 24 campylobacters tested, but not with unrelated bacteria in enzyme immunoassay. Seven antibodies reacting with the boiled antigen in PHA tests were used in serotyping. Strains that showed the same PHA type with polyvalent rabbit antisera could be divided into several antigenically different groups. Similar results were obtained with hybridisations of spleen cells from mice immunised against other campylobacter strains.

Since the monoclonal antibodies function in tests used in preliminary serotyping systems, the results imply that the final serotyping schemes for campylobacters can be defined with monoclonal reagents.

An analogous experiment was carried out as described above, but in this case using the strain **C. fetus** subsp. **venerealis** 14840. Of the 21 clones obtained, eight were positive in PHA tests with saline extracts of whole bacteria; four of these clones also reacted with the polysaccharide and the LPS preparation. Serotyping of 18 **C. fetus** subsp. **venerealis** and **C. fetus** subsp. **fetus** strains with polyvalent rabbit sera showed two different PHA patterns. With the monoclonal reagents, one of these groups of strains could be further divided into four different PHA antigen patterns.

Monoclonal antibody analysis of the surface antigens of Campylobacter jejuni

S. M. Logan and T. J. Trust

Department of Biochemistry and Microbiology, University of Victoria, Victoria, British Columbia V8W 2Y2, Canada

Two approaches were used to isolate hybridoma cell lines producing monoclonal antibodies to surface antigens of **Campylobacter jejuni**. In the first case, spleen cells from mice immunised with formalin-fixed **C. jejuni** VC74 cells were fused with non-synthesising parental myeloma cells and hybridomas that had been selected by means of enzyme-linked immunosorbent assays using 0.2 M glycine HCl (pH 2.2) cell extracts as antigens. Three stable cloned hybridomas were selected which produced antibodies of the IgG class. These antibodies were unreactive in indirect immunofluorescence assays with whole campylobacter cells. The antibodies also failed to react by immunoblotting with a variety of cell fractions, but in radioimmunoprecipitation assays with glycine extracts, and with the periplasmic fraction released from cells by osmotic shocking, all three monoclonal antibodies precipitated a low molecular weight polypeptide triplet. The identity of this triplet antigen is under investigation.

In the second case, mice were immunised with purified flagellin and hybridomas were selected using radioimmunometric assays with the purified protein as antigen. The 12 stable cloned hybridomas selected produced monoclonal antibodies of the IgG class. Using enzyme-linked immunosorbent assays, immunoblotting, radioimmunoprecipitation and indirect fluorescent antibody testing, one antibody was found to recognise a heat-stable determinant common to the surface of thermophilic campylobacter cells and to the type strain of **C. fetus**. The other monoclonal antibodies were specific for flagellin. Analysis of the flagellin with these antibodies indicated that the flagellin was antigenically complex, having a number of determinants exposed on the surface of the native flagellum. One of these surface-exposed determinants appears to be common to the thermophilic campylobacters tested and to the type strain of **C. fetus**. Another surface-exposed determinant was shown to be strain specific, while several determinants appeared to be shared between the flagellins of various other strains of thermophilic campylobacters and **C. fetus**. In addition to three surface-exposed determinants, one monoclonal antibody was specific for a determinant which was not exposed on the surface of the native flagellum.

Monoclonal antibodies against Campylobacter jejuni flagella

D. G. Newell

Public Health Laboratory, Southampton General Hospital, Southampton, UK

Preliminary experiments with the infant mouse model suggest that flagella are important in the pathogenesis of campylobacter infections. Flagella are also antigenic in immunised rabbits and during naturally acquired human infections. Therefore, a number of monoclonal antibodies against flagella have been isolated in order to investigate further the role of flagella in the pathogenesis of campylobacter enteritis and the host immune response.

Balb/c mice were immunised with sarkosyl insoluble outer membrane preparations and boosted with purified flagella from **Campylobacter jejuni** strain 81116. The immune spleen cells hybridised with NS1 cells using poly(ethylene glycol). Twelve hybrid clones producing anti-flagella antibodies were identified using a micro-ELISA technique with sonicates of the flagellated wild-type and an aflagellated variant or purified flagella as the solid phase antigen. Antibody specificity against flagella has been confirmed using immunoblotting of SDS-polyacrylamide gels or radioimmunoprecipitation with ^{125}I-labelled flagella. The cross-reactivity of these antibodies has been investigated with a panel of **C. jejuni/coli** strains, including 17 Penner serotype strains. Several monoclonal antibodies show a broad specificity for all the flagellated strains so far tested; others had varying degres of cross-reactivity. In contrast two clones were specific for strains of the same serotype (Penner 6) as the immunising strain only.

Epitope analysis, using competitive radioimmunoassay with ascitic fluids from the IgG-producing clones, indicates that there are at least four antigenic determinants on the flagella.

Preliminary studies on the passive immunisation of infant mice suggest that some degree of protection against colonisation with **C. jejuni** may be conferred by monoclonal anti-flagella antibodies.

B. SERODIAGNOSIS

Detection of IgG, IgM and IgA anti-campylobacter antibodies by a sensitive radioimmunoassay, and determination of specific IgA size and subclass distribution

F. Mascart-Lemone,* D. L. Delacroix,† M. J. Debisschop,* J. Duchateau,* and J. P. Butzler§

*Department of Immunology and §Department of Microbiology, St Pierre Hospital, rue Haute 322, B-1000 Brussels, Belgium, and †Institute of Cellular and Molecular Pathology, 75 avenue Hyppocrate, B-1200 Brussels, Belgium

Using a pooled antigen preparation (Virion Institute), specific anti-**Campylobacter jejuni** antibodies were detected by a sensitive radioimmunoassay, which was validated for IgG and IgM antibodies through a highly significant correlation between our results and those obtained by complement-fixation. The technique was adapted for determination of specific IgA antibodies using a monoclonal anti-alpha antibody to ensure alpha specificity of the detected antibodies. The **C. jejuni** specificity was confirmed by demonstrating inhibition of binding to the antigen by pre-incubation of positive sera with **C. jejuni** strains, but not with **C. fetus** subsp. **fetus**, **Escherichia coli** or salmonella strains.

Specific IgA antibodies were detected as often as IgG antibodies, though not necessarily in the same sera, and they were more frequent than IgM antibodies. The saliva of three patients having specific IgA serum antibodies were also tested and they all three contained IgA anti-campylobacter antibodies. The specific IgA size and subclass distributions were further analysed. Six IgA positive sera were fractionated by density gradient and tested for total and specific IgA. Whereas polymeric IgA normally represents 13% of total IgA, most IgA anti-campylobacter activity (52-80%) was found to be polymeric. Finally, preliminary results concerning IgA subclass distributions indicated that most anti-campylobacter antibodies are of the IgA_1 subclass.

Our results provide indirect evidence for an intestinal mucosal origin for serum IgA anti-**Campylobacter jejuni** antibodies. The clinical relevance of the detection of these antibodies is being subjected to further study.

Demonstration of serological responses to Campylobacter fetus and Campylobacter jejuni/coli

H. Rautelin and T. U. Kosunen

Department of Bacteriology, University of Helsinki, Haartmaninkatu 3, 00290 Helsinki 29, Finland

Acid glycine hydrochloride extracts prepared from different **Campylobacter fetus** and **C. jejuni/coli** strains were used as antigens in enzyme immunoassay. In general the antisera of rabbits immunised with **C. jejuni/coli** strains showed high reactivity with extracts of different **C. jejuni/coli** strains but low reactivity with those of **C. fetus** strains. Similarly, the antisera of rabbits immunised with **C. fetus** strains showed antibodies to these strains but not to **C. jejuni/coli** strains, indicating antigenic differences between the extracts from **C. fetus** and **C. jejuni/coli** strains. When an extract from **C. jejuni** strain 143483 was used as antigen, most of the **C. jejuni/coli** antisera reacted with it. When this extract was used in human serology, elevated IgM and/or IgG values were found in 73% of patients with campylobacter enteritis. Similar extracts prepared from **C. fetus** strains could be used to detect antibodies in patients infected with **C. fetus**. Several extracts could be used as a combined antigen to screen patient sera.

Alkaline glycine extracts, as employed in complement fixation tests, could also be used in enzyme immunoassay, but a few control sera were reactive. The alkaline extracts showed more bands in SDS-polyacrylamide gel electrophoresis than did the acid ones.

Detection of Campylobacter jejuni and Campylobacter coli serum antibodies using a paper enzyme-linked immunosorbent assay

H. Lior and R. Lacroix

National Enteric Reference Center, Bureau of Bacteriology, Laboratory Center for Disease Control, Tunney's Pasture, Ottawa, Ontario K1A 0L2, Canada

The enzyme-linked immunosorbent assay (ELISA) that we adapted for the detection of human serum antibodies to **Campylobacter jejuni** and **C. coli** has been simplified by substituting the polystyrene microplates for nitrocellulose paper as the solid phase for the binding of antigens.

Extracts of two reference strains of campylobacter used for serotyping (Lior's scheme) obtained by exposing whole cells to glycine-HCl buffer, pH

2.2, were combined and used as antigens. These two extracts were found to give maximum heterologous reactivity with the reference antisera used for serotyping of campylobacters.

Nitrocellulose paper strips previously impregnated with 0.005 ml of antigen extracts were incubated for 3 h at room temperature with serial twofold dilutions of patients' serum. Peroxidase conjugates of antihuman IgG and IgM were applied to the three-times-washed strips for 2 h at room temperature. 4-Chloro-1-naphthol was used as substrate. Positive reactions gave a blue colour within 10 min and end points were read visually. Positive and negative sera assessed by this method were compared with the results obtained with the conventional ELISA using microtitre plates. The antigen-impregnated nitrocellulose paper strips maintained their stability after storage for several months at room temperature. The paper strips can be easily retained as permanent records for reference purposes.

ELISA in the serological diagnosis of campylobacter infections

G. Stanek, A. Hirschl and M. Rotter

Hygiene Institute, University of Vienna, Kinderspitalgasse 15, A-1095 Wien, Austria

A commercially available **Campylobacter jejuni** antigen (Virion, Ruschlikon) and self-prepared phenol-water-extracted lipopolysaccharides from **C. jejuni** and **C. coli** strains were used as antigens for an ELISA. The assay was reproducible, as campylobacter antibody titres did not differ by more than ± one log2 step when sera were tested up to four times.

In tests on 34 sera from children and 14 sera from adult patients with bacteriologically proven campylobacter infections, IgG reciprocal antibody titres of up to 10,000 were found. IgM antibodies could be detected only in low titres. The titres clearly reflect an age relationship. In sera of children aged less than 3 years the titres were low (about 80). In sera from patients aged 4-20 years and more than 40 years, IgG titres were 1280-10,000 and 640, respectively. Additionally, it was established that the maximum titre was attained shortly after the beginning of infection and it remained constant during an observation period of 2 months.

The results indicate that (1) IgG antibody titres against campylobacters increase with age up to 4 years, obviously after repeated antigen contact; (2) IgG antibody titres increase rapidly after a new contact with the antigen and persist over a long period; (3) specific IgM antibodies are detected significantly more often in children than in older persons.

As this type of immune response is typical in people having frequent contact with campylobacters or related antigens, the value of serological tests for diagnosis of recent infections is doubtful. The ELISA procedure therefore seems to offer an advantage in surveys studying the population's immune status.

An ELISA technique for antibodies to **Campylobacter fetus** in bovine vaginal mucus

K. P. W. Gill,* **K. P. Lander*** and P. I. Hewson†

*Ministry of Agriculture, Fisheries and Food, Central Veterinary Laboratory, New Haw, Weybridge, Surrey KT15 3NB, and †MAFF Animal Health Office, Castle House, Newport Road, Stafford, UK

An ELISA technique was compared with the vaginal mucus agglutination test (VMAT) for detecting **Campylobacter fetus** antibodies in bovine cervico-vaginal mucus.

Antigen was prepared from a "sonicated" extract of **Campylobacter fetus** subsp. **venerealis** and the conjugate was a commercial anti-bovine IgG linked to horseradish peroxidase. The substrate was 5-aminosalicylic acid.

The ELISA showed the following advantages in tests on mucus samples from a group of experimentally infected cows:

(1) Positive results occurred earlier than with the VMAT.
(2) More positives were obtained than with the VMAT.
(3) Less sample volume was needed.
(4) It was not necessary to extract the mucus for the ELISA, thus eliminating one stage and making results available more quickly.

Profiles of the serological response to Campylobacter jejuni/coli infection in different situations: normal urban and rural populations, community-wide infection, outbreaks from various sources, occupational groups and so-called sporadic infections

D. M. Jones and J. Eldridge

Public Health Laboratory, Withington Hospital, Manchester M20 8LR, UK

Sera from about 1700 people at risk from **Campylobacter jejuni/coli** infection have been studied using complement fixation, ELISA and bactericidal techniques. The people and situations studied fall into the following groups:

(1) **Individual patients** (a) Individual patients were studied to establish the duration of response as measured by each serological technique and the classes of antibody involved. (b) Individual patients with particular symptomatology, e.g. arthritis, were also studied.
(2) **Normal urban and rural populations** These data form the basis for comparing the response to infection by individuals and groups of individuals.
(3) **Occupational groups** Various occupational groups that handle animals show enhanced levels of antibody, but in general these are not correlated with increased frequency of enteritis.

(4) **Outbreaks** (a) In a number of outbreaks, sera from those with symptoms have been available and these demonstrate the range and variety of antibody response to infection by a single strain of campylobacter. (b) In some outbreaks more than one serotype is involved and some patients may respond simultaneously to infection with more than one serotype. (c) In other outbreaks sera have been examined from a proportion of patients at risk, including those who have had no symptoms; this has demonstrated the prevalence of symptomless infection and also whether the serological response is in any way related to symptoms. (d) On some occasions pre-outbreak sera have been available; these provide unequivocal evidence of infection and show that pre-existing antibody (detected by ELISA or complement fixation) has little effect in terms of protection against clinical illness.

(5) **Sporadic cases** Serological studies of patient contacts can elucidate the likely source of infection by detecting accompanying asymptomatic infections.

ELISA or complement fixation therefore can offer an effective alternative to culture for diagnosis, applicable to sporadic infections and clusters.

Serum bactericidal assay and complement fixation test in the serological diagnosis of campylobacter enteritis: a report on 31 cases

N. Figura,* L. Marri† and A. Rossolini*

*Istituto di Clinica delle Malattie Infettive, Universita di Siena, Via P.A. Mattioli 10, and †Istituto di Microbiologia, Universita di Siena, Via Laterina 8, 53100 Siena, Italy

In this study, the complement fixation test (CFT) has been compared with the serum bactericidal assay (SBA) in the serological diagnosis of campylobacter enteritis. The antigen used in the CFT was the one commercially available, whereas in the SBA the homologous strains had to be used. Twenty-two paired and nine convalescent serum samples (26 from sporadic paediatric cases and five from family outbreaks) were tested. Taking into account the results obtained with both tests, a positivity of 100% was attained:

Methods	No. of positive cases
CFT and SBA	24
CFT only	5
SBA only	2

Sero-conversions were shown in seven cases with CFT and 10 with SBA (in five with both methods). In a control group of healthy children, the CFT detected anti-campylobacter antibodies in 27 (24.5%) of 94 subjects at titres > 1:10 ($P < 0.01$).

The CFT appears a suitable method in the serological diagnosis of campylobacter enteritis. It does not need to be performed with homologous strains and it can detect infections even in cases with negative faeces cultures. The detection of anti-campylobacter antibodies in a relatively high percentage of healthy children may be due to the high prevalence of campylobacters. In fact, in a 2 year study in our area, these micro-organisms were isolated from 16% of children and infants admitted to hospital with enteritis.

Serological response to Campylobacter jejuni infection: evidence for its pathogenic role in indigenous and travellers' enteritis in Bangladesh

M. J. Struelens,* P. Speelman,* R. I. Glass* and S. Lauwers†

*International Centre for Diarrhoeal Disease Research - Bangladesh, GPO Box 128, Dhaka-2, Bangladesh, and †Department of Clinical Microbiology, Free University of Brussels, Brussels, Belgium

The frequency of asymptomatic infection with **Campylobacter jejuni** has raised suspicion about its pathogenic role in Bangladesh. In order to clarify the link between infection and disease we studied the antibody response to **C. jejuni** in infected and non-infected Bangladeshi and foreign newcomers. Sera were examined by complement fixation (CF) (n = 416) and by agglutination (n = 80). **C. jejuni** isolates (n = 57) were O-serotyped by passive haemagglutination. The results were as follows:

		Number in group	No. with CF titre ≥ 1:20		No. with fourfold rise in titre	
Bangladeshi subjects	**C. jejuni**, diarrhoea	53	24	$P = 0.01$	10	$P < 0.05$
	Non-infected, diarrhoea	37	9		1	
Foreign newcomers	**C. jejuni**, diarrhoea	29	17	$P = 0.02$		$P < 0.001$
	C. jejuni, healthy	8	1			
	Non-infected, healthy	28	1			

Antibody responses in the Bangladeshi group occurred only in children aged 6 months to 5 years; CF antibody was not detected in any of 18 healthy Bangladeshi adults. In the foreign newcomers with **C. jejuni** enterocolitis, CF and agglutinating antibodies appeared by the second week of illness and lasted for 3-4 months.

Of 57 isolates from travellers, 78% were typable by Lauwers' scheme:

51% belonged to three serotypes, 27% to 12 other types, all uncommon in Europe. No association was found between a given serotype and clinical presentation or antibody response.

These data show that (a) a commercial complement fixation assay is as sensitive as homologous agglutination for detection of **C. jejuni** antibodies in Bangladesh; (b) frequent antibody response in Bangladeshi and foreign infected patients with diarrhoea supports the pathogenic role of **C. jejuni** in Bangladesh.

Serological diagnosis of Campylobacter jejuni/coli infections

R. Hollander

Staatliches Medizinaluntersuchungsamt, Alte Poststrasse 11, D-4500 Osnabruck, Federal Republic of Germany

The antibody response to **Campylobacter jejuni/coli** infections in man was studied by microagglutination assay against homologous organisms isolated from patients and by complement fixation test (CFT) using a commercially available group-specific antigen of **C. jejuni/coli**. In addition, the CFT was used to determine the antibody titres of healthy blood donors.

Titres of agglutinating antibodies rise within 1-2 weeks of infection to about 1:320 and persist for about 3-4 months. Complement fixing antibodies rise only to about 1:40 but they persist for a long time. Because of the lack of a sero-conversion, the CFT is not suitable for the diagnosis of an acute infection.

Examination of sera from patients with arthritic disorders of unknown cause showed that about 47% (n = 107) exhibited complement fixing antibody titres of > 1:10 against **C. jejuni/coli**. Considering a mean antibody titre of > 1:10 in about 17% of healthy people, 30% of patients possibly suffer from campylobacter arthritis. The persisting complement fixing antibodies allow the diagnosis of reactive arthritis caused by **C. jejuni/coli** to be made, particularly if the causative bacteria are not cultivated.

Evaluation of a commercially available complement fixation test for the detection of campylobacter antibodies

S. Lauwers and R. Bellemans

Department of Microbiology, Akademisch Ziekenhuis, Brussels, Belgium

We evaluated a complement fixation test (CFT) using the antigenic preparations from the Institut Virion AG (Ruschlikon/Zurich) for the detection of **Campylobacter jejuni** and **C. fetus** subsp. **fetus** antibodies.

In order to assess the suitability of the **C. jejuni** antigen as a common antigen, 33 hyperimmune rabbit antisera, prepared against **C. jejuni** reference strains corresponding to 33 different LAU serotypes, were tested. Titres varying from 1/40 to > 1/640 were obtained (normal rabbit sera were negative and the specificity of the **C. jejuni** antigens was satisfactory).

From 171 patients - mostly children - 182 sera were collected at varying time intervals and were also examined. In a first group of 67 patients with a positive **C. jejuni** stool culture, the CFT was positive for **C. jejuni** and negative for **C. fetus** subsp. **fetus** in 34 patients (50.7%). Three sero-conversions were observed. Titres varied from 1/10 (three patients) to 1/160 (one patient); 19 patients had a titre between 1/20 and 1/40. On the same sera, a tube agglutination test (TAT) was performed, using the patient's homologous campylobacter strain as an antigen. The TAT was positive in 38 patients (56.7%). Titres in five of the nine patients with a negative CFT were very low, indicating that the serum specimen was probably taken too early for detection of complement fixing antibodies. The high percentage of negative results with both the CFT and TAT can be explained by the inclusion of a few healthy carriers, many young infants, and the inappropriate timing of some serum specimens.

In a second group of three patients infected with **C. fetus** subsp. **fetus**, the CFT was positive for this organism in all three patients (titres of 1/30, 1/60 and 1/320) and negative for **C. jejuni**.

In a third group of 101 patients suffering from diarrhoea, but with negative **C. jejuni** stool cultures, the CFT for **C. jejuni** was negative in 86 patients (85.1%). Four of the 15 positive CFT results were considered non-specific since both **C. jejuni** and **C. fetus** antigens showed a positive reaction. The remaining 11 patients might have suffered from **C. jejuni** enteritis in the preceding months or **C. jejuni** might have been missed in their stool culture.

The commercially available CFT (Virion), a cheap test which is easy to perform in diagnostic laboratories, proved to be a reliable and useful test for the detction of campylobacter antibodies, particularly in patients with a possible **C. jejuni** enteritis. We routinely test both the **C. jejuni** and **C. fetus** subsp. **fetus** antigens. Sera with positive results for both antigens are considered to be aspecific.

Two years field experience with campylobacter complement fixing antigen

J. Mosimann,* M. Jung,* C. do Vale-Lopez and **V. Bonifas**†

*Institute Virion, CH-8803 Ruschlikon, and †Institute of Microbiology, Chuv, CH-1011 Lausanne, Switzerland

Campylobacter jejuni was isolated from the stools of 210 patients with diarrhoea and abdominal pain. Sera from 152 of these patients were available for serology, most of them as a single specimen. With a newly developed antigen for use in the complement fixation test, which showed a high species specificity and no subtype specificity, we obtained the following results.

Twenty-two sera (14%) were negative, of which 17 were sampled within 8 days of obtaining the positive stool specimen. However, positive results were given by 64 sera obtained under the same conditions. Their titres ranged from 1:10 to 1:240. The high titres (1:60 to 1:240) were observed from the 5th to the 20th day. The most frequent titre observed was 1:30, with 38 sera sampled 3–42 days after the positive stool. Paired sera indicated that sero-conversion was observed in four out of nine pairs. Two patients remained negative. In one case, a titre of 1:60 was observed soon after the positive stool became negative in 20 days. In two cases, the 1:30 titre remained stable. We believe that the antigen used is a convenient diagnostic tool.

Comparison of complement fixation and enzyme-linked immunosorbent assay techniques for the detection of campylobacter antibodies in human sera

J. Oosterom,* S. Lauwers,† J. R. J. Banffer,§ J. Huisman,§ A. E. Busschbach,* R. Bellemans† and C. H. den Uyl*

*National Institute of Public Health, Laboratory for Zoonoses and Food Microbiology, PO Box 1, 3720 BA Bilthoven, The Netherlands; †Department of Clinical Microbiology, Free University, Brussels, Belgium; and §Municipal Public Health Service, PO Box 333, 3000 AH Rotterdam, The Netherlands

During epidemiological investigations in Rotterdam households with a primary **Campylobacter** infection (see abstract on p. 140) serum samples were collected from index cases and both ill and healthy household members. Collection took place approximately 8 days, 22 days and 110 days after first symptoms of enteritis in the initial patient. In total 258 sera were received: from 76 patients on all three occasions, from 14 patients on two occasions, and another two single sera.

Sera were examined using an ELISA technique, in which disintegrated total **Campylobacter** cells were used as an antigen. In addition, examination was carried out by means of a CFT, as described by Lauwers (see

Table 1 Comparison of highest antibody titres with severity of symptoms

CFT									
Titre	0	< 10	10	15	20	30	40	50	> 50
Symptoms									
–	23	–	–	3*	–	1*	–	–	–
+	13	5	–	4	4	4	3	–	4
++	0	1	1	4	2	8	1	–	6
ELISA									
Titre	< 80	80	160	320	640	1280	2500	5000	> 5000
Symptoms									
–	1	6	7	7	6*	–	–	–	–
+	2	1	6	7	6	13	1	–	1
++	–	–	–	2	4	10	4	2	1

*Healthy individual positive in both systems.

abstract on p. 77). Antigens used in the two systems differed both in composition and preparation.

Results showed that highest antibody titres were most frequently found in sera collected after 22 days, but in some cases titres from the first serum samples (8 days) were highest. Only a few of the third set of serum samples showed a positive antibody titre (CFT titre $\geq$ 1:10 and ELISA titre $\geq$ 1:640).

CFT and ELISA indicated identical antibody kinetics in 61 out of 76 sera collected on all three occasions, while in four of these sera kinetics could not be determined using the CFT system because of anticomplementary factors.

Of 258 sera investigated, 141 (55%) were negative using both CFT and ELISA and 75 (29%) were positive using both systems, thus showing identical results in 84%.

Highest antibody titres in the first or second collection serum sample determined by CFT and ELISA were compared to the severity of symptoms experienced by the patients concerned. The results may be tabulated as shown in Table 1.

Session IV

SEROTYPING AND PHAGE TYPING: APPLICATION AND INTERPRETATION

Report on the Session

GENERAL DISCUSSION

The slide agglutination serotyping scheme (Lior) which depends on thermolabile antigens has been extended from the 15 serogroups originally described to 53 (see p. 87). There are further serogroups which are still regarded as provisional. Some of the serogroups are found to be shared by **Campylobacter jejuni** and **C. coli** and some sera react with **C. laridis** strains. An extended biotyping scheme may, with advantage, be used in association with serotyping. Most of the sera used in this scheme require absorption and this is first done with a heated suspension of the homologous strain; however, only about half the sera require further absorption with the heterologous strains. The absorption technique is simple, but as it is essential that each serum is tested initially against the vaccine strains for every serogroup this procedure is best done by staff who are already familiar with it. During the slide-agglutination procedure single colony picks must be used. Freezing and thawing damages the cultures and the strains so treated must be subcultured in broth several times before serotyping. A report from Japan (p. 100) stated that the slide-agglutination reaction involved both heat-labile and heat-stable antigens and that if the formalin-treated suspension which was usually used was replaced by a heated suspension (100 °C for 1 h) the weaker cross-reactions disappeared and the agglutination reaction was clearer. It was implied that the cross-reactions were therefore due to heat-labile antigens.

The scheme from Tokyo could be considered as primarily similar to the Lior scheme, although different reference strains are used (see p. 100). The scheme from Israel (see p. 99), which was able to type about 94% of isolates, also used slide agglutination and initially used living suspensions. Therefore the scheme is essentially similar to that of Lior. Sera were not absorbed and cross-reactions were used to indicate minor antigens and hence sub-types. More recently boiled suspensions have been used and absorptions made. Although repeated passage is needed to avoid auto-agglutination (found in only 4%), the scheme types about 99% of human isolates.

The Lior scheme was used to compare environmental isolates with strains from humans in an area of southern England (see p. 88) and it was found that the range of serogroups was different in the two sources. However, **C. jejuni** serotype 6 was found in water and accounted for 29% of human isolates; the serotype is rare globally. Several serotypes found in water were not found in humans. In Canada the slide-agglutination system was used to elucidate an outbreak in four neonates in a hospital unit (see pp. 87–88). It was shown that each baby had a different serotype and evidence was found that their respective mothers were infected with these serotypes. This agreed with the epidemiological data and cross-infection was discounted.

The scheme using thermostable antigens (lipopolysaccharides) and passive haemagglutination (Penner) now covers 41 serotypes for **C. jejuni** and 18 serotypes for **C. coli** (see p. 90). A supplementary scheme, used only if the strain is found initially untypable, contains 10 and eight serotypes respectively. The diagnostic sera are not absorbed in this scheme and use is made of the cross-reacting antigens in strain discrimination.

A number of presentations were given studying epidemiology and using this Penner typing scheme. In a study in Manchester, England, which covered a one year period, a representative sample of strains was serotyped (p. 90). There was similarity in the range of types found in human infections when compared with those from surface water and farm animals. In the various sources, between 10 and 40% were not typable, the latter figure referring to surface water. A study over a five year period in Southampton, England, showed a pronounced drift in the prevalence of serotypes when 1977 was compared to 1981 (see p. 92); this contrasted with earlier Canadian studies which showed that the same serotypes predominate from year to year. From South Australia it was reported (see p. 93) that for human isolations over a 6 month period generally certain serotypes predominated, but some variations in incidence occur. When isolations from dogs, pigs and chickens were studied, similarities were seen to the range of serotypes in humans.

Three studies reported the comparison between Lior and Penner systems. Considering human isolations in Sweden (see p. 95) it was found that the use of a second system frequently enabled subdivision of types and this applied equally whether the Lior or Penner system was used first. In the CDC Atlanta study (see p. 96) it was confirmed that one system could be used to supplement the other and that by using both together the ability to serotype was increased by between 3 and 5%, the schemes initially typing 95% and 93%. During a milk-borne outbreak in a school in southern England, both systems were used and both identified the epidemic type satisfactorily (see p. 97). Both typing methods also demonstrated that there was a variety of serotypes excreted by the herd of cows that supplied the milk and that these included the "epidemic" serotype.

Studies in Norway and Holland used the Lauwers system to compare the strains from food animals and humans (see pp. 98 and 99). The results in both studies were similar and showed that over 70% were typable. Both studies showed that the serotypes found most prevalent in chickens were the ones occurring most often in humans. This typing scheme, which depends on thermostable antigens and passive haemagglutination, is very similar to Penner's scheme, although different reference strains are used. Nevertheless because both the Penner and Lauwers serotypes depend on the presence of particular lipopolysaccharides the nomenclature of these two schmes could easily be rationalised.

Two alternatives to serotyping were discussed (see pp. 90 and 101). One uses DNA gel electrophoresis and analyses the patterns produced; good agreement with serotyping was reported. The technique had been used on the Penner reference strains and the results were reproducible. A phage-typing technique was presented but some technical difficulties remain unresolved. Nevertheless, using a limited number of phages, almost half the Penner reference strains had been phage typed.

SUMMARY AND CONCLUSIONS

The reports indicate that since the Reading meeting both basic typing schemes (Lior and Penner) have been extended and the epidemiological results show their usefulness. Investigations comparing the two schemes directly are to be encouraged; not only in laboratory studies on reference strains but in different epidemiological settings and geographical areas.

Each of the two basic schemes offers some unique advantages. The Lior scheme uses slide agglutination and techniques for this are regularly used in most clinical laboratories. However, the production of the typing sera requires absorption and this should be done in specialised laboratories already familiar with the technique. This means that as soon as the Lior sera can be made generally available, the scheme should be tested in a number of laboratories, especially in the developing countries. The Penner scheme has the advantage that in general the sera do not require absorption and provided a laboratory has a ready supply of rabbits and the type strains, production of sera should be unimpeded. The identification uses passive haemagglutination, a technique more difficult than slide agglutination but well within the grasp of many laboratories throughout the world. Therefore the use of this scheme in laboratories with the necessary expertise is to be encouraged. Eventually this work will allow comparison of the benefits of each scheme and appropriate recommendations can be made.

For the time being, reference laboratories might use both schemes in view of the reports that one scheme can supplement the other. Such double typing will produce comprehensive information on the direct comparison of both schemes and possibly indicate their relative epidemiological utility. As an alternative, one typing scheme may be combined with an extended biotyping scheme and this combination would also allow greater discrimination of the strains. Examples were the extended scheme of Lior (p. 42) and the resistogram scheme from Preston (p. 42). The latter scheme was used in conjunction with the Penner system to show the heterogeneity of commonly occurring serotypes, e.g. serotypes 2 and 4.

While the antigenic basis for the passive haemagglutination systems has been elucidated, a better understanding of the nature of the antigens involved in the heat-labile system (Lior) is urgently needed. There were some hints in Session III that at least a flagellar antigen (possibly among others) could be involved. Caution is therefore necessary in assuming that slide agglutination systems with live, formalised, or heated suspensions will have similar specificity. Some flagellar antigens are, for example, extremely heat labile.

The development of schemes using minor technical modifications of the two basic schemes seems unnecessary at this stage unless definite benefits can be shown. Even in these circumstances it seems advantageous to use the same set of reference strains as used in the appropriate related scheme (Lior and Penner). Unless this is implemented a proliferation of schemes with different numberings will add to the existing confusion.

B. Rowe

Division of Enteric Pathogens,
Central Public Health Laboratory,
London, UK

D. M. Jones

Public Health Laboratory,
Manchester, UK

Abstracts of Papers Presented

A. SEROTYPING

1. Serotyping by the Lior method (heat-labile antigens)

Serotyping by slide agglutination and biotyping of Campylobacter jejuni and Campylobacter coli

H. Lior, D. L. Woodward, L. J. Laroche, R. Lacroix and J. A. Edgar

National Enteric Reference Center, Bureau of Bacteriology, Laboratory Center for Disease Control, Tunney's Pasture, Ottawa, Ontario K1A 0L2, Canada

The serotyping scheme for **Campylobacter jejuni** and **C. coli** has been extended to 53 serogroups and includes new serotypes identified among cultures from the UK, Yugoslavia, Bangladesh and South Africa. Of 2002 cultures (93%) found to be typable, 1512 strains were isolated from patients with gastroenteritis and 488 strains were isolated from chickens (101), turkeys (55), swine (52) and others (112). Some 156 cultures, 115 from human sources and 41 from non-human sources, were untypable due to roughness. An additional 251 cultures are under investigation as possible new serotypes as belonging to new serogroups. Serogroup 4 was most common among human isolates followed by serogroups 7, 1, 2, 8, 11, 17 and 5. Among non-human isolates, serotype 4 was most common among chicken isolates, serotype 8 among turkey isolates, serotype 20 among swine isolates and serotype 7 was most common among strains isolated from cattle. Although a few serogroups have been so far encountered only among **C. coli** isolates, most **C. coli** belong to the same serogroups found with **C. jejuni** isolates. Among isolates investigated from other countries, 20 different serotypes were identified among cultures from the UK, nine serotypes from Bangladesh, 17 serotypes from Yugoslavia and 16 serotypes among cultures from South Africa. The integration of the serotyping scheme with the new extended biotyping scheme provides more detailed epidemiological information by further differentiating strains belonging to common serogroups.

A pseudo-outbreak of campylobacter enteritis in a newborn nursery

M. A. Karmali,* B. Norrish† and H. Lior§

*Department of Bacteriology, The Hospital for Sick Children, Toronto; †Department of Laboratories, Oshawa General Hospital, Ottawa; and §National Enteric Reference Laboratory, Laboratory Center for Disease Control, Tunney's Pasture, Ottawa, Ontario, Canada

During a 1 week period, four newborns developed campylobacter enterocolitis in a neonatal nursery unit in a 650-bed community hospital. The possibility of cross-infection caused considerable alarm, and raised questions as to whether the unit should be temporarily closed down. A detailed epidemiological investigation suggested that cross-infection was unlikely, and that in all probability the neonates had acquired their infection during delivery from their respective mothers, three of whom were also found to harbour **Campylobacter jejuni** in their stools. This impression was subsequently confirmed by serotyping strains obtained from the babies and their mothers. Each baby was infected by a different serotype (Lior types 4, 7, 11 and 24 respectively). The three culture-positive mothers each had the same serotype as their respective newborns. The fourth mother, who was culture-negative for **C. jejuni**, had serological evidence of infection by the strain isolated from her baby; she developed bactericidal antibodies against her own infant's isolate, but not against the isolates of the three other babies.

Advantage of this outbreak was taken to test the efficacy of the Lior serotyping system in a blind fashion. Up to 10 campylobacter colonies from stools of some of the babies, mothers, and in one case a father and sibling were coded, and sent to the serotyping reference centre without providing information on the source of each culture. The Lior system was able to match correctly by serotype each baby/mother pair of isolates, and it also showed that up to 10 colonies from each stool examined belonged to exactly the same serotype.

Serotypes of environmental and human strains of campylobacter isolated during 1977 and 1978 in Southampton

A. D. Pearson,* H. Lior,† A. C. Tuck* and W. G. Suckling*

*Public Health Laboratory, Southampton General Hospital, Southampton, UK, and †National Enteric Reference Center, Bureau of Bacteriology, Laboratory Center for Disease Control, Tunney's Pasture, Ottawa, Ontario K1A 0L2, Canada

Campylobacter jejuni/coli is widely distributed in the freshwater and marine environment throughout the Southampton area (Table 1). During 1977 **C. jejuni/coli** was detected only in water samples which had evidence of faecal contamination. The presentation detailed the results of biotyping and serotyping (Lior scheme) and compares the prevalence of these markers in the isolates during the same period from human patients in Southampton.

Table 1 Isolation rate of **C. jejuni/coli** from river water and seawater samples in the Southampton area

	No. examined	No. positive	Percentage of samples containing campylobacters (%)
June	45	25	56
July	42	29	69
August	47	6	13
September	25	10	40
October	133	80	60
November	105	59	56
December	74	42	57
Totals	471	251	53

Table 2 A comparison of the prevalence of serotypes of **C. jejuni** strains isolated from environmental and human sources

	Prevalence of serotypes				
	0–1.9%	2–4.9%	5–9%	10–15%	22–25%
Environmental isolates (n = 110)	2; 4; 6;8; 15; 17; 18; 35; 38; 61; 63; 66; 67; NW	23; 28,62; 65		9; NT	64; UI
Human isolates (n = 45)	1,36; 7,38; 8,23; 16,43; 28; 29; 55	1	45; 23; UI	NT	4; 6

NW = new serotype; NT = not typable; UI = under investigation.

RESULTS The prevalence of serotypes in 110 environmental samples is contrasted with that obtained in 45 strains isolated from patients in Southampton during the same period (Table 2).

DISCUSSION The distribution of serotypes in a sample of 110 environmental isolates was different to that of the human series obtained in Southampton during the same period. However, **C. jejuni** serotype 6 biotype III (Lior), which was detected in water, accounted for 23% of the human isolates in the study, yet this type is uncommon in man. Among the 21 serotypes found in the environment, 13 have now been described in association with human infection, five in patients from Southampton. Nine new serotypes have been added to the Lior serotyping scheme as a result of this investigation.

CONCLUSION Some 79 of 110 environmental isolates (63%) have been given an antigenic designation on the basis of the Lior serotyping scheme. Of the serotypes isolated from environmental sources 13 of 21 (62%) have been recognised in association with human infection.

Ingestion of polluted river water and seawater is a mode of transmission for human infection. It is important to assess the relative frequency with which man acquires **C. jejuni/coli** from water prior to making recommendations for the prevention of sporadic cases of campylobacter.

2. Serotyping by the Penner method (heat-stable antigens)

Progress in the development of a serotyping scheme on the basis of thermostable antigens for Campylobacter jejuni and Campylobacter coli

J. L. Penner,* J. N. Hennessy,* R. V. Congi* and A. D. Pearson†

*Department of Microbiology, University of Toronto, Toronto, Ontario M5G 1L5, Canada, and †Public Health Laboratory, Southampton General Hospital, Southampton, UK

A previously described serotyping scheme for campylobacters has been expanded. Forty-two antisera for **Campylobacter jejuni** and 18 for **C. coli** are now used for serotyping isolates of the two species. The thermostable antigens of the isolates are extracted in saline for sensitising sheep erythrocytes for passive haemagglutination titrations of the typing antisera to identify the specificities of the antigens.

In one water-borne outbreak, isolates from six patients were of one serotype and isolates from five others were of another serotype. Two isolates from a contaminated water source were of the same serotype as those from the six patients, thus linking the outbreak to contaminated water. In another outbreak suspected of being caused by contaminated milk, isolates from 29 patients, 10 cattle and one milk sample showed similar reactions in four antisera against closely related serotypes. These reactions were apparently due to cross-reactions as further investigations indicated that the outbreak strain belonged to a new serotype not yet included in the serotyping scheme. In a third outbreak, isolates from patients were found to belong to one or another of two serotypes.

These results suggest that thermostable antigens promise to be useful markers for differentiating isolates in epidemiological studies.

Serotypes and biotypes of Campylobacter jejuni/coli isolated from (a) clinical infections in North-West England during 1982 - a collaborative study by 20 laboratories and (b) non-human sources in North-West England 1982-83

J. D. Abbott, **D. M. Jones**, M. J. Painter, E. M. Sutcliffe and R. A. E. Barrell

Public Health Laboratory, Withington Hospital, Manchester M20 8LR, UK

An investigation was planned to provide information on the epidemiology of sporadic campylobacter infections, which constitute the majority of those in the United Kingdom. During 1982, 1153 cases of campylobacter infection were reported by microbiology laboratories in the ambit of the North Western Regional Hospital Authority of England (with a population of about 4 million); the relevant epidemiological information with the personal details of each patient was obtained by the Region's Infectious Disease Epidemiology Unit. For one month in each quarter throughout 1982, laboratories were invited to send all cultures of **Campylobacter** spp. isolated from human sources to the Manchester Public Health Laboratory. The 311 cultures received during this investigation represented about 25% of the whole year's isolates. Isolates were biotyped by the methods described by Skirrow and Benjamin, and serotyping was carried out by the passive haemagglutination technique of Penner and Hennessy, as shown in the two tables:

Table 1 Serotypes from humans expressed as percentages

Serotype	Percentage	Serotype	Percentage
1,44	10	10	2
2	22	11	2
3	3	19	2
4 (inc. 4,13,16,50)	20	21	2
5	2	23	2
6,7	4	Others	8
8	2	Not typable	17
9,37	3		

Table 2 Serotypes from other sources expressed as percentages

Source	Serotype												
	1,8,44	2	4,13,16,50	5	6,7	9,37	11	19	23	24	27	Others	NT
Water	17	7	9			5		8		5	3	7	42
Cattle	15	23	24				11		9			5	13
Goats	3	31	3	12	2			9	16				25
Sheep	40	15	12		2	4			5			12	10
Chickens	15	5	17	4	7	6		4			12	7	23
Dogs		18	25			3	3	3				23	25

The biotypes and serotypes most commonly associated with human infections were found also to be common among about 900 strains obtained from pond and river waters, cows, dogs, chickens, goats and sheep from the same north-western region.

Major shift in the distribution of campylobacter serotypes identified in 1977 and 1981 from endemic cases in the Southampton area

A. D. Pearson,* J. L. Penner,† R. V. Congi,† A. C. Tuck* and W. G. Suckling*

*Public Health Laboratory, Southampton General Hospital, Southampton, UK, and †Department of Microbiology, University of Toronto, Toronto, Ontario M8G 1L5, Canada

CLINICAL MATERIALS All faecal samples received in the Southampton Public Health Laboratory are cultured routinely for campylobacters on the antibiotic selective medium described by Skirrow. **Campylobacter jejuni** and **C. coli** were isolated from 46 stools in 1977 and 99 stools in 1981. Most of the specimens from which campylobacters were isolated were submitted by general practitioners. No outbreaks or common sources were identified other than within families.

METHODS The strains obtained during 1977 and 1981 were typed according to the scheme described by Penner and Hennessy (extended since publication to include 58 antigenic types). Heat-extracted antigens are used to raise type-specific antisera (non-absorbed) which are titrated by passive haemagglutination against sheep erythrocytes sensitised with the isolate to be typed.

DISTRIBUTION OF SEROTYPES The strains obtained in 1977 were distributed among 11 serotypes, of which seven comprised 65% of the total: the serotype 6,7 was most frequent (28%). The distribution of serotypes in 1981 was very different: 32 serotypes were identified and eight types comprised 60% of the total; serotype 2 accounted for 20%, serotype 4 for 10%, and serotype 6,7 for only 8%. A comparison of the prevalence of serotypes in 1977 and 1981 isolates is shown in Table 1.

Table 1 Prevalence of serotypes isolated from man in 1977 and 1981

	0-3.9%	4-9%	10-19%	20-29%
1977 (n = 46)	13,16,50; 12; 30,51; 37	4; 2; 8; 27; 30	51;	6,7; not typable
1981 (n = 99)	19; 1,44; 2,16; 3; 4,9; 5,30; 6,7,21; 8; 8,11; 8,17; 10,16; 12; 16,50; 21,29; 23; 21,42; 23,36,41; 23,53; 33; 37; 42; 44; 46; 23,36; 24	21; 11; 5; 1; 6,7; not typable	4; 13,16,50	2

DISCUSSION Previous studies have shown that despite the existence of many serotypes of **C. jejuni** and **C. coli**, most clinical isolates belong to relatively few serotypes. A Canadian study showed that the same serotypes predominate from year to year. Our results are in striking contrast with these earlier findings in that: (i) there was a pronounced shift in the distribution of serotypes from 1977 to 1981; (ii) a relatively rare serotype (6,7) was prevalent in both years and was the most common serotype in 1977. This serotype was isolated from water samples in the Southampton area (see abstract on p. 88) and it was reported in association with a water-borne outbreak (see abstract on p. 143).

CONCLUSIONS (1) There appears to be a shift in the distribution of serotypes of **C. jejuni/coli** isolated during 1977 and 1981. (2) Despite detailed clinical and epidemiological investigation of the cases there remains the possibility that the most prevalent serotypes (e.g. 6,7) were from an unidentified outbreak or common source. (3) Possible alternative explanations for the high prevalence of Penner serotype 6,7 during 1977 are: (a) a relatively higher recovery and/or survival of serotype 6,7 as compared to other serotypes; (b) phenotypic variation leading to the expression of the biochemical structural component(s) recognised in the Penner and Lior serotyping schemes as serotype 6; (c) an alteration to the genotype could possibly have been induced by storage and altered growth conditions during isolation or recovery.

Epidemiology of Campylobacter jejuni/coli infections in South Australia. Serotyping of all human and other source isolates from the 1982–83 summer

W. H. Woods,* R. S. Archer* and A. S. Cameron†

*School of Pharmacy and Medical Technology, South Australian Institute of Technology, North Terrace, Adelaide, South Australia, Australia, and †Communicable Disease Control Unit, South Australian Health Commission, Adelaide, South Australia, Australia

Over the period October 1982 to June 1983, 1012 isolates of **Campylobacter jejuni/coli** were serotyped by the procedure of Penner and Hennessy. The valued co-operation of many laboratories has meant that virtually every isolate made in the State of South Australia in that time was included. Isolates were also tested for hippurate hydrolysis and sensitivity to a number of antibiotics.

The majority of isolates (609) were from human faeces submitted to clinical laboratories. Amongst these a total of 66 different serotypes or combinations of reactivity were identified. Certain serotypes predominated, but some common types varied in incidence during the period, suggesting that a similar variation could be expected in isolates from the source(s) of human infection. From veterinary sources 164 isolates were investigated from 16 species, especially dogs, pigs and chickens. Similarities in types prompted a sampling programme from persons, pets and meat in infected households and of raw chicken in shops during February. Over half the 108 campylobacter index cases were still excreting the organism at time of testing and 40 of 283 contacts also carried the organism, although the same serotype was not always identified and some drift of serotype occurred. Campylobacters were isolated from 134 of 259 chicken meat shop samples. A range of serotypes was displayed but the appearance of serotype 37 in chicken meat samples was followed by an increase in incidence of this serotype in cases of human infection.

The serotyping of Campylobacter jejuni and Campylobacter coli isolated from sheep

M. Ansfield and S. J. Duffell

Veterinary Investigation Centre, Block C, Government Buildings, Whittington Road, Worcester, UK

Before the introduction of specialised isolation techniques, **Campylobacter fetus** subsp. **fetus** was the only campylobacter species isolated from sheep. Isolates were relatively few and invariably associated with abortions.

Now the isolation rate has dramatically increased, and **C. jejuni** and **C. coli** together constitute about 50% of all isolates. Unlike **C. fetus** subsp. **fetus**, these species are found readily in a variety of clinical syndromes, e.g. in association with diarrhoea in ewes and lambs as well as in abortions. The clinical significance of **C. jejuni** and/or **C. coli** is not always clear, and biotyping alone is of little help.

The introduction of the passive haemagglutination technique of Penner and Hennessy in 1980 opened the way for further studies, and in 1982 a survey of sheep isolates from England, Scotland and Wales was initiated. Over 200 isolates of **C. jejuni** and **C. coli** have been received and each is being tested against Penner antisera types. Current results are presented.

Isolation and serotypes of animal isolates of Campylobacter Jejuni and Campylobacter coli

D. L. Munroe and **J. F. Prescott**

Department of Veterinary Microbiology and Immunology, Ontario Veterinary College, University of Guelph, Guelph, Ontario N1G 2W1, Canada

Faecal or intestinal material obtained from chickens, cattle and swine were cultured for **Campylobacter jejuni** and **C. coli**. The organisms were isolated from 19.1% of 314 cattle with diarrhoea, 33.9% of 59 pigs with diarrhoea, 27.1% of 398 healthy chickens, 25.2% of 107 healthy dairy cows and 70.1% of 144 healthy pigs. Healthy pigs and chickens were cultured in groups of about 15 animals on separate occasions at slaughter; about 10 cows from each of 10 dairy herds were sampled.

Only **C. jejuni** was isolated from chickens; 92% of the cattle isolates were **C. jejuni**, but 98% of the pig isolates were **C. coli**. With 20 antisera prepared against the most prevalent serotypes found in campylobacter diarrhoea in man, 84% of the **C. jejuni** and 64% of the **C. coli** isolates could be typed on the basis of their thermostable antigens. Some 96% of the chicken isolates, 57% of isolates from cattle with diarrhoea and 60% of isolates from healthy cows belonged to 12 serotypes that also occur most frequently in patients with enteritis, but **C. coli** isolates from pigs belonged to serotypes uncommon among human isolates.

3. Serotyping by the Lior and Penner methods in parallel

The significance of serotyping Campylobacter jejuni

B. Kaijser and E. Sjogren

Department of Clinical Bacteriology, Institute of Medical Microbiology, University of Goteborg, Goteborg, Sweden

Over a period of 12 months in 1978 and 1979, all 198 strains of **Campylobacter jejuni** isolated from patients seeking medical care for diarrhoea at the Department for Infectious Diseases, Eastern Hospital, Goteborg, Sweden, were analysed. Each strain came from one patient. Some 50.5% of the patients were infected outside Sweden, mainly in Europe and northern Africa, and 49.5% were infected in Sweden. The strains were serotyped according to both the Penner system for heat-stable antigens and the Lior system for heat-labile antigens using indirect haemagglutination and direct agglutination respectively. Antisera were prepared by immunisation of rabbits with reference strains obtained from Dr Penner and Dr Lior.

It was found that somewhat different Penner and Lior serotypes dominated in Sweden compared to those reported from North America. The campylobacter serotypes infecting Swedes abroad were also somewhat different from those infecting people in Sweden. The combined Penner and Lior typing showed that each Penner antigen could appear in combination with several different Lior antigens and vice versa. Some combinations, such as Penner 1 and Lior 5 or Penner 18 and Lior 9, were especially common.

The patients were also categorised after clinical symptoms in the following groups: severe diarrhoea/mild diarrhoea, fever/no fever and abdominal pain/no abdominal pain. In pilot studies consisting of 70 out of the 198 patients, some of the antigens were more commonly found in patients with severe clinical symptoms than in others. Thus, regardless of Penner antigen the Lior 9 antigen was more often found in strains from patients with severe diarrhoea and fever than in others. Similar findings were observed for Penner serotype 1 regardless of Lior serotype.

In conclusion we recommend that the two typing systems be used in combination at least for reference laboratories. Except for the apparent significance in epidemiological investigations, serotyping might also be useful in studies on the virulence of individual strains.

Serotyping Campylobacter jejuni/coli by two systems: the CDC experience

C. M. Patton, T. J. Barrett and G. K. Morris

Center for Infectious Diseases, Centers for Disease Control, Atlanta, Georgia 30333, USA

Campylobacter jejuni/coli isolates received at CDC were serotyped by two methods: the Penner method using an indirect hemagglutination (IHA) technique and the Lior method using the slide agglutination technique and absorbed antisera. The isolates were from human and nonhuman sources collected from epidemiologic investigations and special studies. The two systems were comparable in serotyping 425 isolates of campylobacter (Table 1). The Penner and Lior methods typed 95.1% and 93.4% of strains respectively. By using both methods, 98.6% of strains were typable.

Table 1 Serotyping campylobacters from the USA and India/Bangladesh by the Penner and Lior methods

Source	Total tested	Penner			Lior		
		Typable	NT*	UC*	Typable	NT*	Rough*
Human							
USA	116	116	0	0	107	8†	1
India/Bangladesh	142	129	1	12	131	9	2
Animal							
USA	54	54	0	0	53	1†	0
Bangladesh	38	33	4	1	32	3	3
Water							
USA	8	8	0	0	8	0	0
Unknown							
Bangladesh	67	64	1	2	66	1	0
Totals	425	404	6	15	397	22	6

*NT = nontypable, i.e. no reaction in typing antisera (Lior) or no reaction in typing antisera or weak nonreproducible reaction (Penner). UC = unclassified, i.e. reacted in multiple antisera in unexpected combinations which may change from test to test (Penner). "Rough" indicates agglutinated in all or most unabsorbed antisera.

†Nontypable isolates from same outbreak: one serotype by Penner; probably one serotype by Lior.

Although there was not a complete correlation between the serotypes in the two systems, most strains assigned to a single serotype by the Penner method corresponded to one serotype by the Lior method and vice versa. However, multiple serotypes in one system corresponding to a single serotype in the other system did occur, as expected, since the two systems detect different antigens. Lack of complete correlation between the two systems may be useful in epidemic investigations in that strains identical by one system may be subdivided by the other system. The Penner method was the simpler to implement because the system does not require absorbed antisera. However, strains frequently react in more than one antiserum in the Penner system, especially organisms reacting in the 4,13,16,50 complex; test-to-test variation was frequently noted and transient antigens occurred. The Lior method was more difficult to implement because of the need to absorb antisera for antibodies against heat-stable antigens and heterologous activity. However, interpretation of typing results by the Lior method was less difficult, primarily because isolates were more likely to react in only one antiserum. Either method is satisfactory for serotyping **C. jejuni/coli**, but a combination of both methods would be useful for reference laboratories.

A milk-borne outbreak in a school community – a joint medical veterinary investigation

A. D. Pearson,* C. L. R. Bartlett,† G. Page,† J. M. W. Jones,§ K. P. Lander,** H. Lior†† and D. M. Jones§§

*Public Health Laboratory, Southampton, UK; †PHLS Communicable Disease Surveillance Centre, London, UK; §Veterinary Investigation Centre, Winchester, UK; **Central Veterinary Laboratory, Weybridge, UK; ††Laboratory Center for Disease Control, Ottawa, Canada; and §§Public Health Laboratory, Manchester, UK

Six boys reported sick with diarrhoea on 10 November 1982, and the attendances at sick bay reached a peak on 16–17 November. In all, diarrhoea was reported in 29 boys during a 6 week period. The common presenting symptom was headache followed by fever, abdominal pain and diarrhoea. There was usually no nausea or vomiting. Eleven strains of **Campylobacter jejuni** were isolated from 14 faecal specimens. Nine isolates were studied. The predominant outbreak strain was Lior serotype 8/Penner serotype 11. One patient had Lior serotype 4/Penner serotype 2 and two of the patients had strains which typed 8,29 in the Lior scheme; PAGE analysis suggests three type 8,29 to be similar to the outbreak type 8 strains. All the strains were biotype II (Lior).

The results of bactericidal, ELISA and complement-fixation tests on sera from the culture-positive boys showed that most had antibody of at least one sort, but no antibody response was detected in one junior boy and only bactericidal antibody was found in another boy. The prevalence of specific IgG antibody (ELISA $\geq$ 400) among 451 boys sampled 2 months after the peak of the outbreak was 15% (69/451). Infection rates by age group as indicated by serology were: boys aged 9–13, 18% (18/102); boys aged 14–16, 14% (40/276); staff and school community, 21% (12/74).

By means of a questionnaire, diarrhoea was recorded in 32% (34/108) of boys from the Junior school (total 109), 28% (81/290) of boys from the Senior school (total 355) and 14% (24/173) of school staff, monks, nuns, and workers on the school farm. A comparison of milk consumption in 34 Junior school boys who had diarrhoea against 19 controls indicated that there was a significant association between diarrhoea and milk consumption ($P < 0.05$). A comparison of milk consumption in staff and school-workers who had diarrhoea and/or abdominal pain as compared to healthy adults in the school, indicated there was a significant association between diarrhoea and abdominal pain and milk consumption ($P < 0.001$).

Milk was supplied unpasteurised from the school farm. The Friesian herd of 121 adult cows came off the fields to covered yards during October, a few weeks before the outbreak began. All had rectal and quarter milk samples examined for campylobacters by direct and enrichment culture on 30 November. Two litre bulk milk samples were examined between 30 November and 12 January when a further 120 rectal swabs were taken from cattle and cultured for **C. jejuni/coli**. **C. jejuni** was isolated from 25 out of 121 (21%) of animals on 30 November and 31 out of 127 (24%) samples on 12 January. The outbreak serotypes Lior 8 and Lior 4 were the most prevalent (34% and 32% respectively) in the herd. No isolates were obtained from either the quarter milk samples or the 2 litre samples taken between 30 November and 12 January. Inspection of the dairy suggested that faecal contamination of the milk was the most probable route of the infection.

4. Miscellaneous serotyping methods

Serotyping and biotyping of thermophilic campylobacters from man and animals in Norway

G. Kapperud*† and O. Rosef*

*Institute of Food Hygiene, the Norwegian College of Veterinary Medicine, and †Norwegian Defence Microbiological Laboratory, Oslo, Norway

A total of 136 thermophilic campylobacters from patients with gastroenteritis and 350 isolates from domestic (eight species) and wild (seven species) vertebrates from Norway were serotyped on the basis of heat-stable antigens, which were identified by passive haemagglutination using 50 unabsorbed rabbit antisera (Lauwers' serotype scheme).

HUMAN CLINICAL ISOLATES The typable strains (80.1%) fell into 36 different serotypes. The most common serotype was LAU 1, which comprised 7.4% of the typable strains, followed by LAU 2 (5.9%) and PEN 25 (5.9%). A majority of the isolates belonged to **Campylobacter jejuni** biotype 1 (66.3%), followed by **C. jejuni** biotype 2 (20.3%) and **C. coli** (13.4%).

ANIMAL ISOLATES The typable strains (61.4%) fell into 53 different serotypes, 21 of which were encountered among human patients in Norway. The highest proportion of strains showing antigenic relationship to human clinical isolates was detected among poultry (31.2%), followed by wild birds (23.6%), pets (cats and dogs) (18.5%), sheep (14.3%), and pigs (12.1%). Altogether, 86 (24.6%) of the 350 animal isolates tested belonged to serotypes associated with human disease. The serotype and biotype distribution varied considerably between the species of animals examined. Serotypes LAU 1, LAU 2, and LAU 3 dominated with poultry isolates, while LAU 44 was most common among porcine isolates. All porcine isolates were **C. coli**, while **C. jejuni** predominated among domestic and wild birds, sheep and pets. Individual chicken flocks harboured up to nine different serotypes.

Biotype and serotype of campylobacter strains isolated from patients, pigs and chickens in the region of Rotterdam

J. R. J. Banffer

Public Health Laboratory Rotterdam, Schiedamsedijk 95, PO Box 333, 3000 AH Rotterdam, The Netherlands

Campylobacter jejuni strains isolated in the region of Rotterdam were biotyped according to a scheme proposed by Skirrow and Benjamin (1980) and serotyped by passive haemagglutination as proposed by Lauwers (1981) and also by Penner and Hennessy (1980). The antisera for the haemagglutination tests were prepared with prototype strains obtained from Dr Lauwers. The aim was to compare strains originating from three sources: (a) human patients (206 strains); (b) the intestinal contents of pigs from the local slaughterhouse (163 strains); (c) the intestinal contents of chickens at a local chicken slaughterhouse, and from livers sold at poulterer's shops (147 strains).

C. jejuni biotype 1 accounted for 90%, 2% and 84% of strains in categories (a), (b) and (c); **C. coli** accounted for 7%, 98% and 14% of strains respectively.

Serotyping was possible in 77% of the human strains, in 68% of the pig strains, and in 81% of the chicken strains.

The pig strains belonged to 18 serotypes, of which 11 also occurred in humans. The chicken strains belonged to 22 serotypes of which 19 were also represented among human strains.

Statistical testing, using the Spearman rank correlation test, showed that serotypes of higher prevalence in chickens than pigs occurred more often in patients ($r_S = 0.426$; $t = 2.705$; 33 d.o.f.; $P < 0.01$).

Serotyping and biotyping of Campylobacter jejuni from different sources in Israel

M. Rogol and I. Sechter

National Centre for Campylobacter, Government Central Laboratories, PO Box 6115, Jerusalem 91060, Israel

During the year 1982, 560 cultures of **Campylobacter jejuni** isolated in Israel were serotyped with the slide-agglutination method, according to the scheme developed in the Jerusalem Centre for Campylobacter. Among these cultures, 459 were derived from patients with enteritis, 71 from chickens, 28 from cattle and two from dogs.

Some 525 (93.8%) of the cultures were typable with the scheme used, 18 (3.2%) did not react with any of the 58 sera of the scheme, and 17 (3.0%) were autoagglutinable. The percentage of non-typable strains decreased from 8.2% during the first quarter to 1.4% in the last one, thanks to the continuous preparation of new sera.

Among the strains from human sources, the most frequent serotypes were serotype 4 (12.0%), serotype 11 (12.0%), serotype 12 (11.3%) and serotype 9 (5.3%). The serotypes 11 and 12 were frequent during all the seasons. Serotype 4 was found more in the summer. Of the isolates from chicken, 63 (88.7%) were typable. The most frequent serotypes from this source were serotype 11 (46.0%), serotype 28 (11.1%) and serotype 10 (6.3%). Serotype 11 was common in chickens, as well as humans. Of the 28 cultures from calves, 26 reacted with our sera; serotype 4 was prevalent among them and also in humans.

Most of the isolates were biotyped according to the scheme proposed by Skirrow. Of the 422 cultures tested, 79% belonged to **C. jejuni** biotype 1, 15.6% to **C. coli** and 5.4% to **C. jejuni** biotype 2. Biotype 1 was the most frequent in all the sources; **C. coli** was more frequent in calves (28.6%) and chickens (22.2%) than in humans (13.7%) and biotype 2 was not found in calves.

Most of the isolates came from sporadic cases of enteritis. However, some family outbreaks and three community outbreaks were also studied and confirmed by serotyping.

The susceptibility of 103 isolates of **C. jejuni** was tested against 17 antibiotics: 12.6% of the cultures were resistant to erythromycin, 37.9% to tetracycline and 5.8% to ampicillin. Cefazolin and trimethoprim were completely inactive.

Serotyping scheme for Campylobacter jejuni and typing results on the isolates of various origins

T. Itoh, K. Saito, Y. Yanagawa, M. Takahashi, A. Kai, M. Inaba, I. Takano and M. Ohashi

Department of Microbiology, Tokyo Metropolitan Research Laboratory of Public Health, 24-1 Hyakunincho 3-chome, Shinjuku-ku, Tokyo 160, Japan

At the First International Workshop on Campylobacter Infection held at Reading in 1981, we reported that the slide-agglutination test using antigens prepared by formalin treatment and their corresponding antisera was found to be a useful method for serological typing of **Campylobacter jejuni**. By means of this system, 18 serogroups had been identified. Unfortunately, this method was unable to type 50% of isolates from human diarrhoeal cases.

Since then the typing scheme has been further developed to cover an additional 14 types. It now includes 32 different serogroups from TCK 1 through TCK 32. Of the 32 different antisera, 10 of them reacted specifically with their homologous antigens alone; and 22 showed cross-agglutination with some heterologous antigens. Cross-agglutination reactions of 22 antisera were removed by absorbing the antisera with formalin-treated antigens of cross-reacting heterologous antigens, and specific antisera against 32 reference strains have been obtained.

In **C. jejuni**, 420 out of 448 strains of outbreak cases, 735 out of 1156 strains of sporadic cases and 122 strains of animal origin, including four from swine, 41 from cattle, 104 from poultry and 73 from wild birds, were typable specifically by the slide agglutination test. Some 241 strains from sporadic cases and six animal strains were reacted with more than a single antiserum. The common pairs were serogroup 1 and 14, 2 and 12, 3 and 8, 4 and 24 and 20 and 21.

In some cases, these cross-reactions disappeared after treatment of organisms at 100 °C for 60 min. Of 174 strains presenting cross-reaction when formalin-treated antigens were used, 74 (42.5%) of them reacted with a single serum alone, and 82 of them reacted with two or three serotyping sera.

These findings suggest that the antigens involved in the agglutination reaction of **C. jejuni** include relatively heat-stable antigens inactivated by heating at 121 °C for 120 min but not by heating treatment at 100 °C for 60 min and heat-labile antigens which are inactivated by treatment at 100 °C for 60 min. Antisera obtained by immunisation of rabbits with formalin-treated cells were the ones rich in antibodies against relatively heat-stable antigens and the ones with predominance of antibodies against heat-labile antigens.

Our typing system is designed mainly for use in the case of reactions with the relatively heat-stable antigens, and formalin-treated cells used as antigens in the agglutination test were able to be replaced by those treated by heating at 100 °C for 60 min without any essential change in the typing scheme. Heat-treated antigens for the slide agglutination test were preferable to avoid cross-reactions between different types.

B. PHAGE TYPING

Phages of thermophilic Campylobacter spp.: isolation, morphology and utility for typing

A. E. Ritchie, J. H. Bryner and J. W. Foley

National Animal Disease Center, PO Box 70, Ames, Iowa 50010, USA

Practical phage typing of thermophilic campylobacters (**Campylobacter jejuni** and **C. coli**) would aid epidemiological taxonomic studies. For typing, several viruses of known biological activity are needed. Our objective was to acquire several phages and check their typing potential. **C. coli** phages were readily detected and isolated from swine faeces by the lawn/spot method. **C. jejuni** phages, however, were usually lysogenic but could be induced by Mitomycin C discs on lawns (up to 50% of strains tested). **C. coli** phages were of a single morphologic type: 100–120 nm isometric head with a 140–160 nm sheathed tail. **C. jejuni** phages were of at least two types: (a) 60–70 nm isometric head with a 120–140 nm sheathed tail; and (b) 60-70 nm isometric head with a 300 nm non-sheathed "kite" tail. The latter was reminiscent of **C. fetus** phages. Generally, **C. coli** phages did not lyse **C. jejuni** cells and vice versa. However, two **C. jejuni** cultures (rabbit origin) were lysed by **C. coli** phages. Mitomycin induced only **C. coli** phages from these strains.

Interestingly, in two **C. jejuni** strains, Mitomycin induced two different phages. On sequential passage in alternative indicator hosts, one of these phages was lost. Occasionally, mixed "enrichment" cultures (used for detecting indicator hosts) led to prophage induction in the donor rather than in the recipient.

In spite of these unexpected findings, a set of seven phages typed 81% of **C. jejuni** strains, but were inactive against **C. coli**. With another set consisting of five **C. coli** and two **C. jejuni** phages, 23 of 55 (41%) Penner serotype reference strains were typed. The **C. coli** phages typed 15 of 18 strains from swine.

We conclude that recognition and control of the variables noted in this study should help develop practical typing for these organisms.

Session V

PATHOGENESIS

Report on the Session

The papers in this session illustrated a number of features of campylobacter infections in man and animals. They should be read in conjunction with the paper by Black and his coworkers which appears in Session I (see p. 13) and that by Mascart-Lemone and her coworkers which appears in Session III (see p. 71).

INITIAL STAGES OF CAMPYLOBACTER JEJUNI INFECTION IN MAN AND ANIMALS

The first stages of **C. jejuni** infection in man and animals may be considered under two basic headings as follows:

Entry of the organism into the gut

C. jejuni and the other campylobacters are ingested in food and can give rise to disease with as few as 10^4 organisms (Black **et al.**, p. 13). Black and his collaborators have shown that, in their studies, sodium bicarbonate may have enhanced the attack rate, suggesting that gastric acidity may have some protective effect.

Early stages of colonisation

In one presentation (Andremont **et al.**, p. 122) interference with colonisation was reported to occur in gnotobiotic mice when human faecal flora was administered. The reasons for this were discussed but are not entirely clear. Once in the intestine, there seems little doubt that **C. jejuni** localises in areas which allow its survival. In germ-free animals - whether these be dogs, mice or calves - the organisms can be found in the large intestine, which is microaerophilic in such animals (see, for example, Morgan **et al.**, p. 119). Both Dr Lee (Kensington, Australia) and Dr Blaser (Denver, USA) commented on the influence of oxygen on its distribution within the gastrointestinal tract and within the mucosa. It may be that the occurrence of campylobacters in sites such as the stomach, small intestine, appendix and large intestine results in different clinical syndromes and that the pathogenesis of the disease should be defined for each region of the gut.

Once the organism is in the gut lumen, Blaser and Duncan (p. 123) showed that bacteraemia occurred in experimentally infected mice. Similar findings were reported in other animal systems such as chicks (Sanyal **et al.**, p. 122), rabbits (Caldwell **et al.**, p. 114); McCardell **et al.**, p. 128) and calves (Bryner and Warner, p. 120). Bacteraemia could not be demonstrated by Black and his coworkers in healthy human volunteers, and yet both bacteraemia and septicaemia have been documented in man (see Clumeck **et al.**, p. 117). It appears that bacteraemia may be limited by the presence of bactericidal factors in normal human serum (Clumeck **et al.**, p. 117), which may be strain specific in some cases, and by the presence of macrophages in mouse studies (Blaser and Duncan, p. 123). Invasion beyond the basement membrane does not appear to be a major feature of the disease in man, but there is a marked lack of information about the relationships betwen **C. jejuni** and the intestinal tissues in early infection in human disease.

INFECTION AND DIARRHOEA PRODUCTION

The relationship between **C. jejuni** and the intestinal epithelium and the actual mechanism of diarrhoea production was the subject of much discussion. The main features of the relationship appear to be as follows:

Colonisation

The idea that colonisation of the mucus layer of the intestine is important and that **C. jejuni** could exert its effect from this location both in crypts and on the lumenal epithelium was put forward by Lee **et al.** (p. 112) and also in discussion. Proof that it was present in large numbers in the mucus layer was also provided by the photographs shown by McCardell **et al.** in their rabbit study (p. 128).

Adhesion

Adhesion was demonstrated in tissue culture by Newell **et al.** (p. 109), McBride and Newell (p. 110), Lastovica (p. 111) and Cinco **et al.** (p. 112). This adhesion was shown to be associated with different adhesins in the haemagglutination studies of Lastovica and Cinco **et al.** Newell and her coworkers considered that flagella were important - and the presence of serum antibody to flagella in clinical cases of disease suggests that they are indeed involved in some way. There seems to be some doubt, however, about the closeness of the adhesion. Naess **et al.** (p. 111) showed elegant electron micrographs of the relationships between **C. jejuni** and pig brush borders in which the organisms attached much less intimately than does **Escherichia coli**. Other workers, notably McCardell **et al.** (p. 128) and Fauchere **et al.** (p. 124) showed electron microscopic evidence suggesting that adhesion did indeed occur. In discussion, opinion about relevance of adhesion in its strict sense was divided and the term "colonisation" - particularly of the mucosa - was given prominence.

Toxin production

McCardell **et al.** (p. 128) had demonstrated fluid accumulation in the ligated rabbit gut and both McCardell **et al.** (p. 127) and Johnson and Lior (p. 126) demonstrated the presence of toxins. Both groups also showed some identity of the toxic substances with cholera toxin, but there appear to be other toxic substances present as well. Endotoxins are clearly involved in the development of serum antibody responses and may be associated with damage.

Invasion

Invasion of the mucosal epithelium has been clearly demonstrated in some animal infections such as the chick (Sanyal **et al.**, p. 122), the ligated rabbit loop (McCardell **et al.**, p. 128) and mice (Fauchere **et al.**, p. 124). Blaser and Duncan (p. 123) and Fauchere **et al.** provided some evidence that this was more the case of an endocytosis in which **C. jejuni** were taken up by the endocytes than active and destructive invasion.

There is little doubt, however, that invasion by **C. jejuni** is not a major feature of the disease in many of the animal species in which it occurs naturally - in direct contrast to the case of **C. sputorum** subsp. **mucosalis** infections. In the latter, the enterocytes are heavily colonised by the bacteria. The influence which immunity and existing damage have on the ability of **C. jejuni** to invade is not yet clear, but it may be related to region of the gut and to strain as well.

Regional effects

In human volunteers (Black **et al.**, p. 13) and in calves (Morgan **et al.**, p. 119) the large intestine has been affected. The source of the diarrhoea seen in **C. jejuni** infections may be a combination of small intestinal infection with excess fluid production (McCardell **et al.**, p. 128) or paralysis of colonic function and failure of that organ to absorb water due to damage to the enterocytes because of surface colonisation by **C. jejuni**. This mechanism has been shown to be the mechanism of fluid loss in swine dysentery in which **Treponema hyodysenteriae** is conveniently restricted to the large intestine, and does not occur in the small intestine.

Effects on the myenteric plexuses, smooth muscle or intestinal transit times have not yet been described.

SHORT TERM RECOVERY FROM INFECTION

The effect of bactericidal activity in serum accounts quite satisfactorily for the brief and transient nature of most bacteraemias. However, little or no attention has been drawn to the action of neutrophils and macrophages in the gut lumen. These are present in enormous numbers in early infections and may be seen to contain campylobacters in electron micrographs. The fate of these organisms is not known. Lymphocytes are also present in some crypts and may play a part in the immune response.

IMMUNITY TO INFECTION

A number of papers described the immune reactions to infection in man (Black **et al.**, p. 13; Clumeck **et al.**, p. 117). Serum levels of all three classes of immunoglobulin result from infection. The same situation was shown to occur in rabbits (Caldwell **et al.**, p. 114; Ruiz-Palacios **et al.**, p. 115). Ruiz-Palacios **et al.** drew attention to the role of specific secretory IgA in the intestinal response. The involvement of T cells was demonstrated by Rollwagen **et al.** (p. 116).

In practical terms, immunity to reinfection with the same strain was demonstrated in rabbits by Caldwell **et al.** (p. 114) and by Ruiz-Palacios **et al.** (p. 115) and in cattle and sheep by Roberts (p. 121). Roberts also showed that challenge with a different Penner serotype would overcome this immunity.

CONCLUSIONS

The presentations in this session have provided a firm basis of experimental methods and animal infections for the further study of **C. jejuni**. It is of note that infection was described in cattle, pigs, monkeys, chickens and dogs at the First International Workshop and that in this workshop extensive work with mice and rabbits has been added. Infections in sheep and mink (ferrets are more convenient laboratory animals) are also described.

Once it has been decided what actually happens in man – adhesion, enterotoxin production, colonisation of the mucous surfaces, endotoxin production, small intestinal disease or large intestinal disease – the laboratory and animal systems are now available for the investigation of all these mechanisms. In addition, the existence of adenomatous changes such as those of porcine proliferative enteritis associated with catalase-negative campylobacters (Lawson et al., p. 130; Chang et al., p. 131) and the isolation of new types of campylobacter from man should only encourage the search for similar lesions in the human gastrointestinal tract.

D. J. Taylor

Department of Veterinary Pathology,
University of Glasgow Veterinary School,
Bearsden, Glasgow, UK

Abstracts of Papers Presented

A. ADHESION AND ATTACHMENT

The significance of flagella in the pathogenesis of Campylobacter jejuni

D. G. Newell,* H. McBride* and J. M. Dolby†

*Public Health Laboratory, Southampton General Hospital, Southampton, UK, and †Clinical Research Centre, Northwick Park Hospital, London, UK

The function of flagella in the pathogenesis of campylobacter enteritis was investigated using the aflagellate (FLA^-MOT^-) and non-motile (FLA^+MOT^-) variants selected from a wild-type strain, **Campylobacter jejuni** 81116 (FLA^+MOT^+). Biochemical and antigen analysis indicate that the aflagellate variant differs from the wild-type only in the absence of flagella and putative hook protein. The non-motile variant shows biochemical and antigenic identity with the wild-type but is non-motile on motility agar plates and by dark-ground microscopy.

In-vitro studies of adherence using human epithelial cell lines as the target cells are presented on p. 110. These studies indicate that flagella carry an adhesin with a specificity for a receptor expressed on the surface of intestinal epithelial cells. This adhesin is distinguishable from an adhesin(s) on the surface of the bacteria which is detectable using red blood cells as the target cells. Adherence via this second adhesin is inhibited by the presence of active or inactive flagella.

The ability of these three strains to colonise the gastrointestinal tract of the 5 day old infant mouse has been investigated. In this experimental model colonisation is accompanied by attachment of campylobacters to the microvilli of the intestinal epithelial cells. With some strains of **C. jejuni/coli** this attachment is followed by penetration of the epithelium and lamina propria.

The wild-type strain is recovered from the colon, caecum, small intestine or faeces for up to 30 days post-infection. In contrast the aflagellate variant colonises the gut poorly and few, if any, organisms are recovered 7 days after infection. The non-motile variant, however, colonises the gut as efficiently as, if not slightly more efficiently than, the wild type.

These results indicate that motility is not a requirement for virulence in this animal model but that the presence of flagella on **C. jejuni** may confer an advantage in pathogenesis.

In vitro models of adhesion for Campylobacter jejuni

H. McBride and D. G. Newell

Public Health Laboratory, Southampton General Hospital, Southampton, UK

The mucosal surface of the gastro-intestinal tract of man is continually washed by mucus flow. In order for enteropathogenic bacteria to colonise this environment successfully, mechanisms of adhesion have been evolved. Little is known of the mechanisms of attachment utilised by **Campylobacter jejuni**, and in vitro models of adhesion of **C. jejuni** to a variety of target cells have therefore been established.

A defined medium has been developed to encourage the uptake of [^{35}S]methionine by **C. jejuni** and the radiolabelled bacteria were used to measure attachment to cell monolayers or cell suspensions. Additionally, non-motile ($FLA^{+}MOT^{-}$) and aflagellate ($FLA^{-}MOT^{-}$) variants have been selected from a clinical isolate of **C. jejuni** ($FLA^{+}MOT^{+}$) in order to investigate the role of flagella in attachment. All the evidence indicates that, apart from the absence of motility and/or flagella, the variants are identical to the wild-type. On the basis of antigenic specificity with five monoclonal antibodies the flagella of the wild-type and non-motile strains also appear identical.

Comparison of attachment of the variants to epithelial cell line monolayers shows that the aflagellate variant attaches relatively poorly whilst the non-motile variant attaches the most successfully, especially to INT407 cells. This may be explained by the presence of an adhesin on flagella which gives the flagellated organism an adhesive advantage over the aflagellate variant. However, active flagella are obviously a disadvantage, presumably because the contact between the target cell and the motile organism is tenuous. Inactive flagella, therefore, adhere the most efficiently. This attachment is inhibited by a number of sugars, including glucose, galactose, fucose, mannose, N-acetylglucosamine and N-acetylgalactosamine. However, this inhibition may be non-specific as the non-sugar carbohydrate, sorbitol, also inhibits attachment to some degree. Attachment is significantly higher to the fetal intestinal cell line INT407 than to other human epithelial cell lines, which suggests that INT407 cells express a specific receptor for **C. jejuni** flagella.

In contrast to the previous results, the aflagellate strain attaches significantly better than the wild-type or non-motile strains to target cells in suspension, i.e. red blood cells from various animal species and human buccal cells. We therefore postulate the presence of a second adhesin(s) on the surface of **C. jejuni**. The presence of active flagella, and to a lesser extent inactive flagella, hinders the interaction between this second adhesin and the target cell. Further work is in progress to investigate the role of these adhesins in attachment to **C. jejuni** to human intestinal mucosa.

Adhesins on the surface of clinical isolates of Campylobacter spp.

A. J. Lastovica

Department of Microbiology, Red Cross Children's Hospital, Rondebosch 7700, Cape Town, South Africa

Attachment of bacteria to mucosal surfaces is the initial event in the pathogenesis of many infectious diseases in man. A definition of the adhesive molecules on the surface of the bacteria as well as those on the host cell membranes will lead to a better understanding of pathogenic mechanisms of campylobacters.

Twelve strains of **Campylobacter jejuni/coli** isolated from patients at the Red Cross Children's Hospital were examined for the presence of adhesins. These strains were grown under microaerobic conditions on both solid blood agar plates and in liquid medium. The bacteria were harvested at the mid log-phase point in their growth cycle. The strains were negatively stained with phosphotungstic acid and examined under the electron microscope. Pili or fimbriae were not seen in any of the preparations examined.

A convenient, quick and reproducible microtitre assay was developed to test the haemagglutinating properties of the centrifuged test bacteria with erythocytes from man, sheep, rabbit, guinea-pig and mouse. Active haemagglutination was evident at 4 °C, but was also observed at 23 and 37 °C, depending on the particular bacteria/erythrocyte combination tested. In the presence of 0.5% D-mannose, or its analogue, methyl-alpha-D-mannoside, the haemagglutinating activity of three of the bacterial strains was inhibited. The bacteria/erythrocyte haemagglutinated complex formed at 4 °C of two of the bacterial strains eluted when heated to 40 °C. Under the fluorescent microscope, and when challenged with a polyvalent campylobacter antiserum, two of the bacterial strains adhered to epithelial cells. These results indicate the presence of several different adhesins in the cell wall of **C. jejuni/coli**. All of the isolates examined contained at least one plasmid.

Adherence of Campylobacter jejuni to porcine brushborders

V. Naess, A. C. Johannessen and T. Hofstad

Departments of Microbiology and Immunology and Pathology, The Gade Institute, University of Bergen, Bergen, Norway

Brushborders were isolated from the small intestines of freshly slaughtered pigs. **Campylobacter jejuni** strains NCTC 11168, NCTC 11392 and NCTC 11351 were grown in a biphasic culture system consisting of Brucella agar plates covered with 10 ml Brucella broth, both containing FBP supplement. The plates were incubated at 42 °C under microaerobic conditions for 3 days.

Mixtures of washed bacteria and brushborders were incubated for 15, 30 or 60 min at 37 °C on rollers. The brushborders were harvested and washed to remove non-adherent bacteria, and were studied by phase contrast microscopy, various light microscopic staining techniques, indirect fluorescent microscopy and scanning and transmission electron microscopy.

The ratio of bacteria to brushborders had to exceed 100:1 for any apparent adherence to take place. There were no differences in the number of adherent bacteria between 15 and 60 min of incubation. The best way to visualise the adherence was by scanning electron microscopy. The bacteria were found to adhere to both the brushborders and the adjacent cell fragments.

This in vitro model can be used to study the nature of the receptor on the brushborder and the adhesin on **C. jejuni**.

Studies on the adhesive properties of campylobacters

M. Cinco, E. Banfi and D. Crotti

Institute of Microbiology, University of Trieste, via A. Fleming 22, 34127 Trieste, Italy

The adhesive properties of 12 strains of **Campylobacter jejuni** and two of **C. coli** of human origin were studied. They were firstly tested for haemagglutination of human, guinea-pig, horse, sheep and rabbit erythrocytes.

Only a few of the tested strains gave any agglutination of human and guinea-pig erythrocytes at high concentrations of bacteria. On the other hand, the campylobacter isolates tested on jejunum cell cultures all showed adhesion to a significant extent.

Further experiments employing known inhibitors of adhesiveness to identify the receptor(s) involved gave evidence of one L-fucose-specific and heat-stable adhesin.

Campylobacter jejuni as a mucosa-associated organism: an ecological study

A. Lee, J. O'Rourke, M. Phillips and P. Barrington

School of Microbiology, University of New South Wales, PO Box 1, Kensington, New South Wales 2033, Australia

The surfaces of the gastrointestinal tract of most animals so far examined have been found to be colonised by large numbers of bacteria. Through a period of evolution with their natural host, these microorganisms have adapted specific mechanisms for association with mucosal surfaces.

A constant feature of the majority of organisms colonising intestinal crypts of animals, including rodents, dogs and guinea-pigs, is that they have a spiral morphology. We have been successful in culturing many of these organisms using campylobacter-selective agar and microaerophilic growth conditions.

Campylobacter jejuni has a spiral morphology similar to that of organisms previously described as inhabitants of intestinal crypts and has been isolated from normal rodents, dogs and pigs. Recent observations with the scanning electron microscope of mice colonised by **C. jejuni** have revealed sheets of **C. jejuni** on the colonic surface. Thus it was considered possible that **C. jejuni** is a mucosa-associated bacterium specifically adapted to the mucus environment of the intestinal surface. This hypothesis was tested in gnotobiotic Balb/c mice maintained in plastic isolators. Mice were inoculated by the orogastric route with 0.1 ml of a thick suspension (10^{10} per millilitre) of a human isolate of **C. jejuni** for three successive days. Animals were killed after 1 week and tissue specimens were examined.

The caecal crypts of control mice were seen to be empty while the crypts of all mice inoculated with the campylobacter culture were seen to be full of the characteristic spiral bacterium.

The majority of the caecal crypts in the inoculated mice were colonised by large numbers of campylobacters, while only a few of the crypts in the ileum or colon were colonised and by smaller numbers. This suggests a preferential colonisation of the caecal mucosa by these bacteria.

Germ-free mice and specific pathogen-free mice with no normal mucosa-associated flora were also inoculated with campylobacter cultures and the caecal mucosa examined for bacteria. The colonisation of crypts was not as heavy as in the gnotobiotic animals. Variable colonisation of intestinal crypts depending on the microbial status of the animal has been observed with another microaerophilic spiral organism isolated from the rodent gut which appears to colonise similar locations to **Campylobacter** spp. Due to its characteristic morphology this organism can be recognised in conventional animals, where it preferentially colonises the small intestine compared to the gnotobiotic mouse or rat where the colon and the caecum are heavily colonised. This observation may be relevant to the finding that **C. jejuni** causes crypt lesions in the small bowel of conventional dogs while caecitis and colitis are found in gnotobiotic dogs.

The reasons for this association with intestinal surfaces and the apparent affinity for mucus have been investigated. Spiral bacteria in other systems have been shown to be well suited to a viscous environment due to their characteristic motility. This property would be an ecological advantage in the mucus-filled crypts. Therefore videotapes of cultures of campylobacters and other gut organisms in solutions of varying viscosity were observed and the motility measured using a planimeter. Cultures of a human campylobacter isolate and the spiral inhabitant of intestinal crypts were shown to be better able to move in solutions with a viscosity approximating intestinal mucus compared to other gut organisms.

These findings confirm the hypothesis that **C. jejuni** is a surface-associated organism in the mouse intestine. Histological studies in normal dogs suggest that the same will be found with these animals.

The ability of this organism to associate closely with intestinal surfaces may have important consequences with respect to the pathogenicity of human infection, which has been poorly understood to date. Histologic sections of biopsies from patients with severe infection show an acute colitis with inflammatory infiltration of the lamina propria, with crypt abscesses being an important feature. Recently, inflammatory bowel disease has been studied in a colony of marmosets; destruction of crypt abscesses was found to be associated with colonisation by **C. jejuni**.

SUMMARY **C. jejuni** colonises the mucus layer and crypts of the intestinal mucosa of mice. Factors that influence surface association are (a) oxygen tension and (b) adaptation to mucus, e.g. motility. The site of crypt colonisation may vary depending on the ecological milieu of the gut.

HYPOTHESIS Colonisation of mucus is an essential step in the pathogenesis of campylobacter infection. Attachment may not be necessary.

B. IMMUNITY AND IMMUNE RESPONSE

Development of an adult rabbit model of campylobacter infection suitable for testing immune responses to disease

M. B. Caldwell, R. I. Walker and S. D. Stewart

Naval Medical Research Institute, Bethesda, Maryland, USA

We found that the removable intestinal tie-adult rabbit diarrhea (RITARD) procedure is a simple way of establishing **Campylobacter jejuni** infection which mimics human disease. With this procedure 64% of 55 rabbits receiving 1.35×10^9 c.f.u. of **C. jejuni** developed loose, mucus-containing stools after an incubation period of 1-6 days. The mortality rate was 53% of animals challenged and death was always preceded by diarrhea. Blood cultures were taken daily from 30 rabbits during the 4 days after challenge. All challenged animals had at least one positive culture. Pathological examination of eight symptomatic rabbits showed abnormal intestinal histology in seven of the eight.

After we determined that campylobacter enteritis could be produced in rabbits with the RITARD procedure, we tested the hypothesis that RITARD-induced infection could be prevented by previous colonization induced by gastric inoculation with live organisms. Gastric feedings containing 5×10^8 c.f.u. were administered to 16 animals. The mean number of days for which these rabbits were rectal swab positive for **Campylobacter** was 15.8 $\pm$ 2.4. No rabbit had diarrhea during this period.

After 21 days these rabbits, along with 10 unexposed control animals, were challenged with 1×10^9 c.f.u. of **Campylobacter** administered by the RITARD procedure. The mean number of days for which immune rabbits were rectal swab positive for **Campylobacter** was 1.3 $\pm$ 2 compared to 9.8 $\pm$ 3.7 days for control animals. Four previously exposed animals were not protected from colonization and three of these developed diarrhea.

Blood cultures were obtained 24 h after gastric feeding or the RITARD procedure. Seven of 16 rabbits sampled were, following gastric feeding, bacteremic with **Campylobacter**. Following the RITARD challenge, none of 10 immune rabbits were bacteremic compared to all of five non-immune animals.

The serum IgG response was measured by whole cell indirect ELISA. The mean serum IgG response 3 weeks after the gastric feeding was 1593. Since the mean titre of the four animals not protected was 2848, there may be no correlation between serum IgG response and protection.

Systemic and local immune response in experimental campylobacter infection

G. M. Ruiz-Palacios, Y. Lopez-Vidal, A. B. Lopez-Vidal, J. Torres and S. Rubio

Instituto Nacional de la Nutricion, San Fernando y Viaducto Tlalpan, 14000 Mexico, D.F., Mexico

In order to study the development of immunity to **Campylobacter jejuni**, adult New Zealand rabbits were challenged with 10^4 and 10^8 colony forming units (c.f.u.)/ml of **C. jejuni** strain INN-1-79, using the RITARD model. Diarrhoea was induced with 10^4 c.f.u. on day 7 in 10 of 14 rabbits (70%) and with 10^8 c.f.u. on day 3 in 100%. Shedding of **C. jejuni** started on day 1 post-infection in all rabbits receiving 10^8 c.f.u., but only in 70% receiving 10^4 c.f.u. Both groups shed **C. jejuni** for 5 days. Animals from both groups were rechallenged with 10^8 c.f.u. on weeks 5-8. None developed diarrhoea nor shed campylobacter in faeces.

ELISAs were developed to detect serum and intestinal tissue immunoglobulins. A serum antibody response was observed in all rabbits receiving 10^8 c.f.u. The mean log IgG titres were 2.45 ± 1 on the second week, and peaked on the third with mean titres of 3.2. IgG declined by week 8 to 2.9 ± 0.42. IgM antibodies were detected earlier, 3-7 days after the first challenge, with mean log titres of 2.9 ± 0.4 in rabbits receiving 10^8 c.f.u.; titres remained high after 8 weeks. IgG and IgM titres were more than one log lower in rabbits receiving 10^4 c.f.u.

Monomeric IgA anti-**C. jejuni** somatic antigen was not detected with either 10^8 or 10^4 c.f.u. Interestingly, secretory IgA was detected in high titres the first week after challenge in all animals receiving 10^8 c.f.u., and only in two of eight animals (25%) receiving 10^4 c.f.u., and in low titres. After rechallenge with 10^8 c.f.u., there is an increase in IgG, IgM and secretory IgA (S-IgA) titres in animals first challenged with 10^8 c.f.u.

No increase in IgG or IgM was seen after rechallenge of rabbits that first received 10^4 c.f.u., but a striking rise in specific S-IgA titre was observed after rechallenge in this group, reaching levels similar to those of the other groups.

No statistically significant difference in antibody levels from intestinal tissue was observed between the groups receiving 10^8 or 10^4 c.f.u. As compared with controls, levels of non-specific immunoglobulins from intestinal tissue rose when animals were challenged and rechallenged. Intestinal non-specific S-IgA levels increased four times with rechallenge, but IgG levels remained essentially the same.

Specific intestinal anti-**C. jejuni** antibodies were not detected in the control group. Specific IgG was not detected after the first challenge, and levels were very low after rechallenge.

In contrast, specific S-IgA was detected following the first challenge, and levels were seven times greater after the second challenge.

From the data presented, the following conclusions may be drawn:

(1) Using the RITARD model, an immune response to **C. jejuni** infection could be induced.

(2) The size of the inoculum seems to influence the triggering of different immune responses. While relatively low doses trigger a mainly secretory response, high doses trigger intense systemic and local responses.

(3) Both low and high doses seem to confer protection against a second infection by a homologous strain.
(4) S-IgA plays a definitive role in the immunity of campylobacter infection.
(5) The detection of specific S-IgA in serum should be taken with caution and requires further investigation. There is normally little S-IgA in the serum of human beings and other animals. However, levels could rise under certain circumstances such as hepatobiliary obstruction, lactation, metastasic cancer of the liver, and cirrhosis, where there is an impairment of the uptake and transport of dimeric IgA in the liver to the biliary tract. It is therefore possible that an exaggerated production of S-IgA in the intestine of immunised animals could saturate temporarily the hepato-biliary shunt that normally clears this immunoglobulin, leaking it to the bloodstream.

T-cell responses to Campylobacter jejuni in rabbits

F. M. Rollwagen, M. B. Caldwell and S. D. Stewart

Naval Medical Research Institute, Bethesda, Maryland, USA

Lymphoid cells from rabbits which had recovered from experimental **Campylobacter jejuni** infection were tested for their capacity to proliferate in vitro to either nonspecific or specific stimuli. Proliferative respones were assessed using lymphoid cells from spleen, Peyer's patch and mesenteric lymph node, tested against sonicated isolates of **C. jejuni** and **C. fetus**. Nonspecific proliferative responses to concavalin A (Con A) were also evaluated. No differences were observed in the proliferative response to any concentration of Con A. Spleen, Peyer's patch, and mesenteric lymph node cells from infected rabbits proliferated in response to nanogram amounts of **C. jejuni** sonicates. Proliferative responses were reduced by 90% when boiled antigens were used as stimuli.

Specificity testing revealed several patterns of response among the three lymphoid cell populations tested. Heteroclitic responses (higher response to nonrelated antigen) were observed only with spleen cells. Peyer's patch cells from some rabbits responded specifically, whereas those from other rabbits responded to all three antigens. Mesenteric lymph node cells proliferated in response to all antigens. No response was observed when lymphoid cells from uninfected rabbits were used.

T-cell lines were established from proliferating cultures of spleen, Peyer's patch or mesenteric lymph node cells. Such T-cell lines are currently being tested for specificity and capacity to provide help, as well as surface phenotype, using flow microfluorometry. T-cell clones will provide a sensitive means of analyzing bacterial components for their ability to induce T-helper cells. Suitable cell components may then be tested as vaccine candidates.

C. HUMAN INFECTION

Natural immunity against Campylobacter jejuni infections

N. Clumeck, M. Steens, Ph. Vandeperre and J. P. Butzler

Infectious Disease Unit, St Pierre Hospital, and WHO Collaborating Centre for C. jejuni, 322 rue Haute, 1000 Brussels, Belgium

Most serotypes of **Campylobacter jejuni** are destroyed by normal human serum (NHS). It has previously been shown that the bactericidal reaction of NHS involved both the complement classical pathway and IgM antibodies. In order to determine the specificity of these antibodies and their acquisition during life, sera were obtained from healthy volunteers and children, who had no previous history of infection and whose ages ranged from 2 weeks to 40 years. Normal cord human sera and sera from children aged 0-6 months were not bactericidal to five serotypes of **C. jejuni** (serotypes 1, 2, 3, 6, 34), whereas bactericidal activity was found in the age group 6-12 months. Cross-absorptions of NHS with heat-boiled **C. jejuni** belonging to the 12 most frequently isolated serotypes and with a mutant of **Escherichia coli** 0111 (J_5 mutant) showed that bactericidal antibodies, although serotype-specific, were absorbed by the J_5 mutant. This study suggests that bactericidal immunity against **C. jejuni**, which appears early in life, may occur without previous contact with campylobacters and may be directed against an antigen (core of colipid) shared in common by Enterobacteriaceae and **C. jejuni**.

Serum bactericidal deficiency in Campylobacter jejuni septicaemia

N. Clumeck, M. Steens, Ph. Vandeperre and J. P. Butzler

Infectious Disease Unit, St Pierre Hospital, and WHO Collaborating Centre for C. jejuni, 322 rue Haute, 1000 Brussels, Belgium

Septicaemia due to **Campylobacter jejuni** is a rare clinical feature during acute gastroenteritis. It has been shown previously that nearly all **C. jejuni** isolated from blood cultures were destroyed by pooled normal human serum (NHS). In order to test the hypothesis that septicaemia results from a host deficiency, rather than a higher virulence of some strains, bactericidal activities of NHS and of serum from three patients with a septicaemia due to serotypes 3, 34 and Pen 10, were compared. Bactericidal activity of serum was studied by incubating **C. jejuni** (5×10^5 c.f.u./ ml) from 24-hour cultures with 80% fresh serum for 60 min at 42 °C. In all cases, strains isolated were sensitive (less than 10% survival) to NHS and resistant to autologous serum (patient's serum). In two cases the bactericidal deficiency was specific to the infecting strain, in one case with low circulating IgM antibodies; the deficiency extended to all serotypes tested.

These preliminary results may explain (1) the rarity with which **C. jejuni** septicaemia occurs and (2) the role played by host deficiencies in **C. jejuni** septicaemia.

A comparison of host susceptibility and pathogenicity of Campylobacter jejuni infection in school children and adults during three outbreaks

A. D. Pearson* and J. R. Davies†

*Public Health Laboratory, Southampton General Hospital, Southampton, and †Public Health Laboratory Service, 61 Colindale Avenue, London NW9 5EQ, UK

This presentation compared the outbreak curves and host responses in pupils and staff from three boys' boarding schools. The outbreak in School I (see Hoskins an Davies, p. 14; Wilson **et al.**, p. 143) was a point source milk-borne outbreak of short duration (about 1 week), whereas those in School II (see Pearson **et al.**, p. 143) and School III (see Pearson **et al.**, p. 88) lasted for 6-8 weeks. A comparison of attack rates and subclincal infection rates as determined by questionnaire analysis and prevalence of antibody (bactericidal, ELISA, and CF) is presented in Table 1.

Table 1 Comparison of three outbreaks of **C. jejuni** in schools with pupils aged 9-18

Host response	School I	School II	School III
Isolation rate for **C. jejuni**	36/41 (88%)	17/34 (50%)	11/24 (79%)
Attack rates			
Diarrhoea	295/784 (38%)	234/625 (37%)	115/464 (25%)
Pain	28%		
Infection rate (subclinical)	15%		
Serotype			
Lior scheme	7	6 and 39	4 and 8
Penner scheme	4 complex (13,16,43,50)	6 and 58 (40)	2 and 11
Bacteriocidal antibody (Penner)		6, 40 and 41	
Source and serotypes at source	Milk (Lior 7) Cattle (Lior 7)	Water tank (Lior 6/ Penner 6)	Cattle faeces (Lior 4 and 8)

TRANSMISSION FACTORS The milk-borne outbreak in School I was from a point source and showed no evidence of secondary cases. Multiple serotypes were detected in the outbreaks in Schools II and III. The long duration and multiple peaks suggest that these were intermittent source outbreaks. Epidemiological studies suggest there was faecal contamination of the water and milk supply (birds and cattle). The dilution factors for these outbreaks were very high, which suggests that infection took place with a low dose of **C. jejuni**. The milk from outbreak III was cooled in a 2600 litre tank. The capacity of the main water tank in outbreak II was 12,000 gallons (54,500 litres). There were high attack rates as measured by prevalence of diarrhoea. This indicates a high susceptibility to **C. jejuni** of these populations of school children and adults. Antibody studies indicate that in outbreak I there was a 15% subclinical infection rate. Analysis of the questionnaires suggests that abdominal pain could occur in the absence of diarrhoea.

CONCLUSIONS (1) A low or very low dose of **C. jejuni** may infect children and adults who drink contaminated water or milk. (2) A high infection rate (81%) occurred in outbreak I when diarrhoea, abdominal pain and subclinical infection were considered as markers of infection. (3) We would suggest that the detailed investigation of an outbreak requires questionnaire analysis; blood samples from cases and controls; and strain recovery from cases, transmission vehicles, and potential sources/reservoirs. (4) Areas for further investigation are (a) determination of whether there are differences in infecting organisms or host response in patients with abdominal pain or subclinical infection as compared to that in cases with diarrhoea; (b) B and T cell responses in the three types of infection; (c) whether variations in growth conditions affect the ability to cause infection.

D. NATURAL AND EXPERIMENTAL C. JEJUNI ENTERITIS IN ANIMALS

Natural and experimental campylobacter infection of calves

J. H. Morgan, G. A. Hall, D. J. Reynolds and K. Parsons

ARC Institute for Research on Animal Diseases, Compton, Newbury, Berkshire, UK

NATURAL INFECTIONS Faeces from normal and affected animals from 44 outbreaks of calf diarrhoea were examined for various microbiological agents, including **Campylobacter** spp. The results were as follows:

	C. fetus subsp. fetus	C. jejuni/coli
Normal calves (n = 364)	13%	25%
Diarrhoeic calves (n = 463)	20%	34%
Significance	$P < 0.01$	$P < 0.01$

In 11 outbreaks campylobacters were detected in $\geq$ 60% of cases, but these outbreaks were associated with other recognised bovine pathogens. In none of these outbreaks were campylobacters the **only** agent present in the majority of cases.

EXPERIMENTAL INFECTIONS Five gnotobiotic calves were orally infected with mixtures of **C. jejuni** and **C. coli**. Clinical effects were similar in all calves. After a prodromal period of fever and blood in faeces, a mild illness with prolonged excretion of soft mucoid faeces occurred. Maximum effects were observed 2-4 weeks after inoculation and were associated with persistent high-level excretion of campylobacters ($\pm 10^9$ c.f.u./g).

At postmortem, campylobacters were found in high numbers (10^6-10^{10}) in the large intestine and tonsil, in moderate numbers (10^3-10^6) in the small intestine and in low numbers ($\pm 10^3$) in the abomasum, mesenteric lymph node and gall-bladder.

Blood cultures remained negative.

Pathological examination revealed haemorrhage and tissue debris on the mucosal surface in early cases, and petecchial haemorrhages in the colonic mucosa in animals examined after 2-4 weeks.

Microscopically there were foci of mixed inflammatory cells in the lamina propria, with exfoliation of abnormal and degenerating enterocytes.

Campylobacters were observed by immunoperoxidase staining on the mucosal surface, in the epithelium and lamina propria and colonising glands. Intra-epithelial organisms were associated with lesions in some sections.

CONCLUSIONS We have found only a small (albeit statistically significant) difference in isolation rate between normal and diarrhoeic animals, no outbreak associated with pure campylobacter infection, and only mild disease in experimentally infected gnotobiotic calves. We therefore consider that these results fail to prove that **C. jejuni/coli** or **C. fetus** subsp. **fetus** are important in the pathogenesis of calf diarrhoea. Further work with experimental infections and pathology of experimental infections is required.

Experimental infection of neonatal calves with thermophilic campylobacters

J. H. Bryner and D. P. Warner

National Animal Disease Center, PO Box 70, Ames, Iowa 50010, USA

Milk-borne human enteric campylobacteriosis is a subject of public health concern. This study was designed to expand the knowledge of the dynamics of infection, pathogenesis and carriage of **Campylobacter jejuni** and **C. coli** in neonatal calves [1].

Three colostrum-deprived and five colustrum-fed calves aged 3-10 days were infected orally with 4.8×10^9 c.f.u. per calf of **C. jejuni** strain 958 (ovine aborted fetus source) in commercial milk replacer (500 ml). Within 3 h, **C. jejuni** was cultured from peripheral blood of the calves; bacteremia persisted at least 42 days in one calf, 28 days in two, 14 days in one, and shorter periods in the others. The organism was cultured from feces of two calves at 8 weeks, four calves at 7 weeks, and shorter periods in the remainder.

Three colostrum-deprived calves, aged 4-8 days, were infected orally with 10^{10} c.f.u. per calf of **C. coli** strain 1380 (swine aborted fetus) in commercial milk replacer (500 ml). Within 2-3 h, **C. coli** was cultured from all calves and bacteremia persisted up to 6 days, 4 days, and 2 days. The organism was cultured from feces of each calf up to 21 days.

We conclude that bacteremia in clinically normal lactating cows with **C. jejuni** or **C. coli** might play a role in milk-transmitted human enteric campylobacteriosis.

REFERENCE

1. D. P. Warner and J. H. Bryner. Experimental **Campylobacter jejuni** and **Campylobacter coli** pathogenesis in neonatal calves. Submitted to the American Journal of Veterinary Research.

Infection and reinfection experiments with Campylobacter spp. in domestic animals

L. Roberts

Veterinary Investigation Laboratory, Mill of Craibstone, Bucksburn, Aberdeen AB2 9TS, UK

Chickens (1-7 days old) proved susceptible to experimental enteric infection after oral inoculation with campylobacter isolates from a wide variety of sources (human, animal and bird isolates). More than 90% of dosed chickens became infected, except for those dosed with **Campylobacter laridis**, in which only half of the dosed birds became infected. Infected birds remained clinically healthy. There appeared to be site differences with respect to colonisation for different isolates, and campylobacters were commonly recovered from the livers of dosed birds. Although all isolates used had been minimally passaged, chickens were dosed with fresh faeces from human cases of campylobacter enteritis (**C. jejuni** biotype 1 isolated) in order to overcome the possible loss/failure to express virulence determinants in vitro. As in other chicken experiments, all inoculated birds became colonised, but again no frank clinical disease was produced.

Both sheep and cattle (from newborn to over 1 year old) were reared campylobacter free and have been experimentally infected with a wide range of **Campylobacter** spp. from human, animal and bird sources. The only strain which did not colonise after oral inoculation was **C. laridis**. Infected animals remained clinically healthy and passed a variable amount of mucus in faeces, although stool consistency was usually not altered. The main histopathological changes were enlargement of Peyer's patches and the mesenteric lymph nodes.

Reinfection experiments were also carried out in sheep and cattle. This work indicated the presence of resistance homologous but not heterologous challenge, with typing based on the passive haemagglutination technique of Penner and Hennessey for heat-stable antigens.

Pathogenesis of Campylobacter jejuni diarrhoea in an experimental model

S. C. Sanyal, P. K. B. Neogi, K. M. N. Islam and M. I. Huq

International Centre for Diarrhoeal Disease Research - Bangladesh, GPO Box 128, Dhaka-2, Bangladesh

A diarrhoea model for **Campylobacter jejuni** has been developed in 36-72 h old chicks using 40 strains isolated from samples of watery diarrhoea and six strains from samples of bloody mucoid diarrhoea. Since the detection of diarrhoea in chicks is difficult, the volumes of fluid in the gut of 288 birds fed with live **C. jejuni** in doses of 10^3-10^6, compared with 183 saline-fed controls, was taken as the criterion for diarrhoea.

The peak incidence of diarrhoea (81%) and maximum volume of fluid in the gut occurred on the fifth day. Watery diarrhoea was common irrespective of whether a strain had been isolated from a simple or a bloody enteritis case; however, four of the isolates from the latter group caused mucoid rather than bloody diarrhoea in chicks. Five of the controls developed non-specific diarrhoea.

The organism multiplied in the ileum and probably the colon by 2-5 log and caused systemic invasion in 47% of the chicks on the fifth day. Histopathology revealed no change in the intestinal mucosa of chicks having watery diarrhoea, but those with mucoid diarrhoea showed exudative changes with necrosis, and in one the organism was seen inside the epithelial cells. Change of electrolyte composition of diarrhoeal fluid was limited to an increase in K^+ concentration.

This study indicates that oral administration of **C. jejuni** in infant chicks is followed by multiplication of the organism in the ileum, and perhaps the colon, causing mainly watery diarrhoea and occasional inflammatory changes in the gut. There is local and/or systemic invasion and the nature of the diarrhoeal fluid indicates elaboration of enterotoxic substance(s).

Microbial antagonisms of human faecal flora against Campylobacter jejuni: a study in gnotobiotic mice

A. Andremont, F. Leonard, F. Goldstein, Y. Pean, S. Pequet and C. Tancrede

Microbiologie Medicale, Institut Gustave-Roussy, 94800 Villejuif, France

Microbial antagonism within the lumen of the colon is one of the possible mechanisms of resistance to colonisation by enteropathogenic micro-organisms. In vivo antagonisms exerted by human faecal microflora against **Campylobacter jejuni** have been studied in gnotobiotic mice. Germ-free C3H mice were maintained in plastic isolators. They were exposed to complex human faecal flora and strains of **C. jejuni** sequentially in this or the reverse order. We had previously shown that bacterial equilibria present in the original microflora were readily transferred to the mouse intestine both quantitatively and qualitatively. Microbial antagonisms were also reproduced and could be studied in this animal model.

A strain of **C. jejuni** given alone to the mice was eliminated within a week after the addition of the faecal microflora of a healthy volunteer. Similarly **C. jejuni** was rapidly eliminated when given to mice previously exposed to the same faecal microflora. When faeces of patients with acute campylobacteriosis were given to germ-free mice, the animals shed **C. jejuni** at a concentration of 10^8 c.f.u./g of faeces over several weeks without showing any clinical signs or any colonisation of the biliary tract. Post-treatment faecal flora of these patients could also be colonised by the strain of **C. jejuni** isolated during the acute phase of the disease. The persistence of this modification of the barrier effect against **C. jejuni** might be due to the antibiotic treatment, inasmuch as erythromycin sharply decreased the resistance to colonisation by **C. jejuni** of the faecal flora of a healthy volunteer.

Characteristics of Campylobacter jejuni bacteremia in experimentally infected mice

M. J. Blaser and D. J. Duncan

Infectious Disease Section, VA Medical Center, and Division of Infectious Diseases, University of Colorado School of Medicine, Denver, Colorado, USA

We have previously observed that bacteremia is common following **Campylobacter jejuni** infection of adult mice. We now report results of studies concerning the characteristics of intraluminal to bloodstream transit of **C. jejuni** and observations on clearance mechanisms.

After atraumatic oral application of **C. jejuni**, passage through the stomach results in a 1-3 log decrease in organisms reaching the small intestine. A high proportion of intraluminal **C. jejuni** pass directly through the small intestinal wall. The liver, but not the spleen, is the major clearance site. Ten minutes after oral ingestion of 10^7-10^8 **C. jejuni**, blood contains 10^3-10^4 c.f.u./ml, a concentration that remains relatively constant for 1 h. This bacteremia is transient and by 12-24 h post-dose the bloodstream is again sterile. After intravenous **C. jejuni** administration, clearance is similarly rapid. Liver and spleen clear organisms equally per gram of tissue. High intravenous doses (10^7 c.f.u. or higher) result in fecal excretion of **C. jejuni** which is associated with biliary carriage. Biliary carriage is related to peak **C. jejuni** concentration in the bloodstream. Poisoning macrophage function with silica resulted in decreased bloodstream clearance of **C. jejuni** after intraperitoneal challenge. These studies document the natural course of bacteremia after oral **C. jejuni** infection in an animal model and suggest that reticuloendothelial macrophage function is an important host defense against orally ingested **C. jejuni**.

Experimental infection with Campylobacter jejuni in germ-free or monoxenic mice

J. L. Fauchere, M. Veron, A. Pfister and A. Lellouch-Tubiana

Laboratoire de Microbiologie, Faculte de Medecine Necker-Enfants Malades, 156 rue de Vaugirard, 75730 Paris cedex 15, France

The purpose of this study was to develop a model of intestinal infection with **Campylobacter jejuni** in adult germ-free or monoxenic mice. It was found that the gut of all mice orally inoculated with 10^8–10^9 bacteria was colonised. Diarrhoea was usually observed from day 4 to day 10. **C. jejuni** was isolated from faeces over a period of 50 days. It was possible to estimate the number of intraluminal bacteria (duodenum and ileum, 10^2–10^5; colon, 10^8–10^{10}) and that of mucosa-associated bacteria (duodenum and ileum, about 10^3; colon, 10^3–10^7), as expressed by the number of bacteria per gram of gut. The proportions of total bacteria which were mucosa associated were about 50% in the duodenum, 1–10% in the ileum and 0–1% in the colon. **C. jejuni** was regularly isolated from Peyer's patches and mesenteric lymph nodes until the 10th day, irregularly between day 10 and day 15, but never later. **C. jejuni** was never found in spleen or liver.

Histopathological studies did not demonstrate any significant damage to the intestinal mucosa. However, bacterial adherence on the mucosa and bacterial endocytosis by enterocytes were observed by electron microscopy.

In this study, **C. jejuni** invasiveness of tissues was apparently related to attachment to the intestinal mucosa, endocytosis by enterocytes and bacterial growth in the intestinal lymphoid system, without invasiveness of the reticular endothelial system. Experiments with monoxenic mice demonstrate that accompanying flora do not invade the intestinal lymphoid system.

Animal-passaged, virulence-enhanced Campylobacter jejuni causes enteritis in 6-day-old mice

S. U. Kazmi,* B. S. Roberson,* and **N. J. Stern**†

*Department of Microbiology, University of Maryland, College Park, Maryland 20742, and †Meat Science Research Laboratory, Agricultural Research Service, US Department of Agriculture, Beltsville, Maryland 20705, USA

An animal model mimicking human campylobacteriosis was developed. Intraperitoneal injection of adult BALB/c mice with **Campylobacter jejuni** suspended in 2.5% mucin or 2.5% iron dextran lowered the LD_{50} from about 10^{10} colony-forming units (c.f.u.)/ml to 10^5 c.f.u./ml. The strains required three passages in animals to become lethal. Iron dextran and mucin enhanced virulence and lethality when given with **C. jejuni**, but development of signs and the rate of killing were faster when iron dextran was injected 3 h before inoculation. Of strains tested by intragastric or intraperitoneal injection without iron dextran or mucin, only one isolate from chicken meat was found lethal, killing only some animals. All intraperitoneal injected mice developed the following signs 1–10 days post-injection: loose watery feces with mucus, ruffling of fur, lethargy and labored breathing. Deaths occurred from one to several days post-injection. Dead animals had enlarged spleens and normal livers, but the large intestines were swollen and filled with loose fecal material and sometimes blood.

Six-day-old mice were challenged by intragastric intubation of 2×10^9 c.f.u. animal-passaged, virulence-enhanced isolates of **C. jejuni**. All animals developed signs of infection by day 5, manifesting severe diarrhea with increasing mucous discharge and reduced weight gain. Diarrhea continued for 8 days, after which all animals recovered. This research provides a means of determining mechanisms of pathogenesis and of assessing virulence potentials of isolates.

Natural and experimental campylobacter diarrhoea in mink

B. D. Hunter* and **J. F. Prescott**†

*Department of Clinical Studies and †Department of Veterinary Microbiology and Immunology, Ontario Veterinary College, University of Guelph, Guelph, Ontario, Canada

RANCH 1 Of 900 mink, 160 litters were affected. Kits still in the nestboxes were normal, but developed diarrhoea at 3–4 weeks of age, after they had left the nestboxes and were eating solid food. The kits were febrile and produced a yellow-green mucoid diarrhoea, with flecks of blood. Many showed tenesmus; a few developed rectal prolapse. Some died of exposure. Adult mink were unaffected. Erythromycin in the feed stopped the outbreak. A total of 75 kits died and 25 became "poor doers" and were killed. The only viral or bacterial pathogen identified was **Campylobacter jejuni**: this was found only in affected animals.

RANCH 2 Some 300 of 1800 litters were affected at 3–4 weeks of age, when they went on solid feed. Clinical signs were more severe than in Ranch 1. The outbreak was stopped with erythomycin. Only affected mink were infected with **C. jejuni**; no other viral or bacterial pathogens were identified. The rancher developed severe diarrhoea. **C. jejuni** was recovered from chicken waste fed in the ration.

EXPERIMENTAL INFECTION Four **C. jejuni**-free mink of 7 weeks of age were infected orally with 10^8 **C. jejuni** obtained from the abortion outbreak described by Prescott **et al.** (p. 129). At 48 h after infection faeces became loose and at 72 h they contained mucus and blood. Mink were killed at 96 and 120 h after infection. Four control mink were unaffected.

PATHOLOGICAL EXAMINATION Gross examination of naturally and experimentally infected mink showed that the small intestine contained excess yellowish fluid. The colonic mucosa was hyperaemic, with the mucoid contents flecked with blood. Multiple 1 mm focal or 1 mm wide linear ulcers were observed in the region 2 cm distal to the ileal-colonic junction.

Histopathological changes in naturally infected mink were as follows:

(a) the colonic mucosa was thickened; (b) there was an inflammatory cell infiltrate in the lamina propria and the submucosa; (c) numbers of crypt and goblet cells were decreased; (d) the remaining crypt cells were dilated, often with cellular and inflammatory debris (crypt abscesses); (e) multiple areas of mucosal ulceration were observed; (f) lesions occurred consistent with ulcerative colitis. Experimentally infected mink showed similar but milder histopathological changes.

E. TOXIN PRODUCTION

Toxigenicity of Campylobacter jejuni and Campylobacter coli associated with human enteritis

W. M. Johnson and H. Lior

National Enteric Reference Center, Bureau of Bacteriology, Laboratory Center for Disease Control, Tunney's Pasture, Ottawa, Ontario K1A 0L2, Canada

The pathogenic mechanism by which **Campylobacter jejuni** provokes a diarrhoeal response in humans has not yet been well established. Whereas the invasive potential of **C. jejuni** has been demonstrated in experimental animals, several investigators have recently attempted to establish the possibility of a classic enterotoxin- and/or cytotoxin-mediated diarrhoea. We have performed extensive enterotoxigenicity studies on both stool filtrates from **C. jejuni** positive stools and culture filtrates from clinical isolates of **C. jejuni**. All toxigenicity studies were performed using standardised tissue culture and immunological assays. Cell lines used to monitor the presence of enterotoxins and/or cytotoxins include monkey kidney cells (Vero), mouse adrenal tumour cells (Y-1) and Chinese hamster ovary cells (CHO). Suckling mouse assays were performed for detection of heat-stable (ST) type enterotoxins. More than 50 culture-positive **C. jejuni** stool filtrates from children with gastroenteritis unrelated to other recognised enteric pathogens have been tested to date. In stool filtrates, both heat-stable (80%) and heat-labile (60%) factors reactive in Vero and CHO cells have been detected. Neutralisation studies were performed using standardised antitoxins to cholera toxin, **Escherichia coli** heat-labile enterotoxin (LT) and **Clostridium difficile** cytotoxin. Cytotoxin active against Vero cells has been demonstrated in filtered culture supernatants of over 60% of **C. jejuni** strains grown in biphasic medium. This cytotoxicity is heat-labile and has also been detected in culture filtrates from clinical strains of **C. coli**. In addition to cytotoxin, over 80% of the **C. jejuni** strains tested have been shown to produce a heat-stable cytotonic response in Vero, Y-1 and CHO cells. No fluid accumulation could be demonstrated in suckling mouse assays of the heat-labile cytotoxic or heat-stable cytotonic preparations. Over 50 clinical isolates have been characterised for toxigenicity to date and studies are presently in progress to delineate any relationship of serotype, biotype and toxicity of the **C. jejuni** strains being investigated.

Isolation and partial characterization of toxin produced by *Campylobacter jejuni*

B. A. McCardell,* J. M. Madden* and E. C. Lee†

*Food and Drug Administration, Washington, District of Columbia 20204, and †The Catholic University of America, Washington, District of Columbia 20064, USA

An enzyme-linked immunosorbent assay (ELISA) based on binding to cholera toxin antibody was used to screen cell-free supernatants from 12 strains of **Campylobacter jejuni**. Seven of the eight clinical isolates, one animal isolate and one food isolate were positive, suggesting that these strains produced a toxin immunologically similar to cholera toxin. Although all cell-free supernatants were negative in the Y-1 mouse adrenal cell assay, protein from ammonium sulfate-treated supernatants caused cell rounding. Cell-free supernatants and concentrates heated at 90 °C for 15 min and tested by the suckling mouse assay produced no fluid accumulation in the intestines of mice. However, cell-free concentrates were positive in the rabbit skin permeability test and caused fluid accumulation in rabbit ileal loops.

An affinity column (packed with Sepharose 4B conjugated to purified anti-CT IgG via cyanogen bromide) was used to separate the toxin from cell-free concentrates. Rounding of Y-1 mouse adrenal cells produced by campylobacter toxin was eliminated by treatment with trypsin or preincubation with cholera antitoxin. However, rounding was unaffected by heating at 56 °C for 30 min, 60 °C for 10 min or 100 °C for 10 min. The campylobacter toxin showed partial identity with cholera toxin by slide gel immunodiffusion. Molecular weight was estimated by gel filtration to be 68,000 daltons.

Studies on the pathogenicity of *Campylobacter jejuni* in experimental mouse campylobacteriosis

E. Kita,* N. Katsui,* Y. Yanagase† and S. Kashiba*

*Department of Bacteriology, Nara Medical College, 840 Shijyocho, Kashihara City, Nara 634, and †Department of Bacteriology, Hyogo College of Medicine, Nishinomiya City, Hyogo 633, Japan

Invasive ability and other pathogenic features of 96 clinical isolates of **Campylobacter jejuni** were tested for in the mouse uterus. Ten of the isolates showed a strong ability to invade the epithelium of the uterus and induce transient bacteremia. Fifty-four of the isolates showed no invasion but produced fluid accumulation in the lumen of the uterus. The remaining 32 isolates possessed both activities but to a much lesser degree.

Invasive activity paralleled that of serum resistance of three strains. The most invasive strain had significant amounts of membrane proteins with high molecular weight as well as heat modifiable protein analysed by SDS-PAGE. Both invasive ability and production of fluid accumulation might be involved in the mechanism(s) of campylobacter enteritis. A study is being undertaken to clarify the relationship of the pathogenic mechanisms in the uterus to those of the gastrointestinal tract.

Evidence for multiple pathogenic mechanisms in infections with Campylobacter spp.

B. A. McCardell,* **J. M. Madden,*** J. W. Bier,* E. C. Lee† and H. L. Dallas*

*US Food and Drug Administration, Washington, DC, and †US Naval Medical Research Institute, Bethesda, Maryland, USA

Despite the recent detection of a toxin immunologically similar to cholera toxin in cell-free supernatants of **Campylobacter jejuni** and **C. coli** cultures, there is evidence to suggest that **Campylobacter** spp. possess another mechanism of pathogenicity. The injection of 18 h **C. jejuni** and **C. coli** cultures into permanently ligated rabbit ileal loops produced fluid accumulation and morphological changes in intestinal tissue that are typical of an acute enteritis. The morphology observed in hemotoxylin and eosin stained intestinal sections was similar to that produced by **Shigella dysenteriae** 1, and contrasted sharply with the milder changes brought about by cholera toxin. Injection of **C. jejuni** cultures into rabbit ileal loops also resulted in a transient bacteremia which was detectable within 10 min and lasted 2-3 h. At 24 h no bacteria were detected in the blood, but organisms were isolated by swabbing the interior of kidney, liver or spleen and by culturing fluid from intestinal loops. No bacteria were cultured from the lung or heart. Scanning electron micrographs of intestinal tissue showed a thick accumulation of mucus mixed with bacteria. In a few areas where mucus was absent, campylobacters were observed attached to villi. Immunoperoxidase staining of intestinal tissue sections demonstrated the presence of **C. jejuni** in the cells of the epithelial layer and the lamina propria. The pathological tissue effects and the local invasion of intestinal tissue have yet to be correlated with a specific cytotoxin and/or adherence factor.

F. MISCELLANEOUS INFECTIONS

An outbreak of Campylobacter jejuni abortion in mink

B. D. Hunter,* J. R. Pettit† and J. F. Prescott§

*Department of Clinical Studies, Ontario Veterinary College; †Veterinary Laboratory Services, Ontario Ministry of Agriculture and Food, Ottawa; and §Department of Veterinary Microbiology and Immunology, Ontario Veterinary College, University of Guelph, Guelph, Ontario, Canada

An outbreak of **Campylobacter jejuni** abortion occurred on a mink ranch with 1059 breeding females. Other animals on the ranch (15 cattle, 15 coon hounds, 15 silver foxes and a small flock of Pekin ducks) were unaffected. The owner fed the mink on a self-mixed ration of cereal base, tripe, liver, eggs and chicken offal, which he also supplied to three other mink farms, which were unaffected. A small pond adjacent to the well supplying drinking water to the mink was thus thought to be the source of infection, rather than the food.

The first abortion was observed on 10 April 1982 and dead mink kits were discarded. In late April and early May many mink went off feed for 2–3 days and developed grey mucoid droppings, occasionally tinged with blood. The mink remained bright and there were no adult deaths. Of the affected mink, 189 aborted (18% of breeding females) but another 312 failed to produce kits and probably included animals which resorped rather than aborted fetuses. Erythromycin in the feed appeared to prevent further abortions. **C. jejuni** Penner serotype 37 was isolated from all aborted fetuses in large numbers, from mink faeces, and from duck faeces, but not from other sources including the feed. Some people on the ranch developed diarrhoea but refused to be cultured.

Campylobacter jejuni mastitis in cows: bacteriology and pathology

K. P. Lander* and A. Baskerville†

*Ministry of Agriculture, Fisheries and Food, Central Veterinary Laboratory, New Haw, Weybridge, Surrey, and †PHLS Centre for Microbiology and Research, Porton Down, Salisbury, Wiltshire, UK

In experiments designed to assess the possible significance of **Campylobacter jejuni** as an infection of the bovine udder, the following observations were made:

(1) Six of seven strains of **C. jejuni**, from various sources, were able to induce mastitis in cows.
(2) Thirty-two udder quarters of 22 cows developed mastitis following the intra-mammary inoculation of small numbers of **C. jejuni**.

(3) Three udder quarters of 12 cows developed mastitis following twice daily immersion of the teat ends in broth cultures of **C. jejuni**.
(4) The induced disease varied from acute severe mastitis with systemic effects to mild inapparent disease.
(5) **C. jejuni** multiplied within infected udder quarters and the organisms were excreted in the milk.
(6) The duration of bacterial excretion varied from 3 to 73 days.
(7) The bacterial excretion rate varied from high (> 5×10^5 per ml) to low and intermittent.
(8) The peaks of bacterial excretion usually preceded the peaks of clinical and pathological signs.
(9) Histopathology of severely affected quarters showed a moderate inflammatory reaction without necrosis but with large areas of alveoli heavily infiltrated with polymorphonuclear leucocytes.

It was concluded that naturally occurring cases of udder infections with **C. jejuni** were quite possible. Such cases could result in the contamination of raw milk with large numbers of **C. jejuni**.

A comparison of the behaviour of Campylobacter sputorum subsp. mucosalis in gnotobiotic piglets and tissue culture

G. H. K. Lawson, A. C. Rowland, E. McCartney, M. Rajasekhar and G. Fraser

Department of Veterinary Pathology, University of Edinburgh, Royal (Dick) School of Veterinary Studies, Edinburgh, UK

Intracellular vibrioid bacteria are a constant feature of the lesions of porcine intestinal adenomatosis (PIA) and from such tissues **Campylobacter sputorum** subsp. **mucosalis** can often be isolated in large numbers. Despite this close association between bacteria and abnormal cells, the part played by the organism in the induction of the lesions remains unclear. Repeated studies, in which pigs of different immunological status have been exposed to abnormal mucosa containing intracellular vibrioid bacteria, have largely failed to result in disease or the establishment and multiplication of subsp. **mucosalis** in the mucosa.

Exposure of gnotobiotic piglets to subsp. **mucosalis** results in both oral and intestinal colonisation by the organism, but cultural, histological and ultrastructural studies have failed to show the presence of intracellular bacterial parasitism or adenomatosis, and these experiments have shown that the bacteria, which may be isolated from the mucosa, are a "spill-over" of luminal colonisation. Neither intercurrent rotavirus or cryptosporidial infection modifies the relationship between cells and vibrios, nor does the presence of a defined aerobic intestinal bacterial population interfere with the luminal colonisation by subsp. **mucosalis**.

In contrast to the observations made in gnotobiotic piglets, in tissue culture subsp. **mucosalis** attaches readily to a number of cell lines. The response of such cells in vitro depends on their type, but in those to which bacteria attach readily intracellular multiplication takes place and may persist for long periods.

Campylobacter hyointestinalis, a possible cause of proliferative enteritis in swine

K. Chang, **G. E. Ward**, C. J. Gebhart and H. J. Kurtz

College of Veterinary Medicine, University of Minnesota, St Paul, Minnesota 55108, USA

Campylobacter hyointestinalis, a previously undescribed, catalase-positive, hydrogen sulfide-positive organism, was isolated from 67% of swine with lesions of proliferative enteritis. **C. hyointestinalis** could be distinguished from other campylobacters from swine (**C. sputorum** subsp. **mucosalis** and **C. coli**) using antiserum produced in rabbits in agglutination and fluorescent antibody tests.

Fluorescent antibody tests showed **C. hyointestinalis** to be present in 29 of 29 naturally occurring lesions of proliferative enteritis in high numbers deep within crypt epithelial cells in the ileal region. In contrast, **C. sputorum** subsp. **mucosalis** was found in only 24 of 29 lesions of proliferative enteritis and was associated more commonly with necrotic debris and surface mucosa. Using an immuno-peroxidase test, 14 of 15 specimens from lesions of proliferative enteritis showed high numbers of **C. hyointestinalis** in crypt epithelial cells, whereas only three of 15 showed **C. sputorum** subsp. **mucosalis** in crypt epithelial cells.

Sera from adult swine in Minnesota showed a high proportion (> 95%) of positive titers (range 1:16 to 1:250) to both **C. hyointestinalis** and **C. sputorum** subsp. **mucosalis**. Antibody to both these organisms is apparently transferred via the colostrum, because neonatal pigs had titers similar to dams. This antibody decays to undetectable levels by 4 weeks of age.

Efforts to reproduce proliferative enteritis in swine with pure cultures of **C. hyointestinalis** and **C. sputorum** subsp. **mucosalis** together or separately were unsuccessful.

Campylobacter hyointestinalis: a possible cause of [illegible] proliferative enteritis in swine

K. Chang, G. E. Ward, C. J. Gebhart and H. J. Kurtz

College of Veterinary Medicine, University of Minnesota, St Paul, Minnesota 55108, USA

Campylobacter hyointestinalis, a previously undescribed catalase-positive, hydrogen sulfide-positive organism, was isolated from 67% of swine with lesions of proliferative enteritis. C. hyointestinalis could be distinguished from other campylobacters from swine (C. sputorum subsp. mucosalis and C. coli) using antiserum produced in rabbits in agglutination and fluorescent antibody tests.

Fluorescent antibody tests showed C. hyointestinalis to be present in 20 of 29 naturally occurring lesions of proliferative enteritis, in high numbers deep within the crypts and in epithelial cells in the ileal mucosa. In contrast, C. sputorum subsp. mucosalis was found in only 14 of 29 lesions of proliferative enteritis and was located more commonly with necrotic debris and surface mucosa. Using the immunoperoxidase test, all 11 specimens from lesions of proliferative enteritis showed high numbers of C. hyointestinalis in crypt epithelial cells, whereas only three of 11 showed C. sputorum subsp. mucosalis in crypt epithelial cells.

Sera from adult swine in Minnesota showed a high proportion ([illegible]) of positive titers (range 1:16 to 1:320) to both C. hyointestinalis and C. sputorum subsp. mucosalis. Although antibody to both these organisms is apparently transferred via the colostrum because pigs had titers similar to their dams, this antibody decayed considerably by 4 weeks of age.

Efforts to reproduce proliferative enteritis in swine with pure cultures of C. hyointestinalis and C. sputorum subsp. mucosalis together or separately were unsuccessful.

Session VI

EPIDEMIOLOGY AND SURVIVAL EXPERIMENTS

Report on the Session

SUMMARY

This report considers the new data made public at this meeting and the epidemiological questions which deserve exploration before the 1985 meeting.

The investigation of outbreaks has indicated that water, raw milk and poorly cooked food, especially poultry, are sources and vehicles of infection. This knowledge provides a rationale on which to base preventive measures. The application of serotyping methods to the study of outbreaks gave the participants an insight to both the need for accurate designation of antigenic structure and the requirements for additional markers with which to trace **Campylobacter jejuni/coli.** Investigation of sporadic infection by case control studies indicates that risk factors vary with age, locality and season. The study of reservoirs, specifically water and environmental samples including mud, wild birds and animals, flies and foodstuffs established that there is often contamination with C. **jejuni/coli** where serotypes are common to those found in man. Campylobacter is confirmed as a common cause of travellers' diarrhoea.

Studies in the developing countries indicate that infection occurred more commonly in young children and frequently in association with other gastrointestinal pathogens. There were no case control studies from the developing world, no data that related serotyping markers with source or mode of transmission and no new evidence of secondary infections. This absence of case to case transmission in developing countries or developed countries confirms the validity of the existing public health measures stated in 1981 by the Public Health Laboratory Service:

(a) Precautions relevant to enteric infection should be maintained for the duration of symptoms, i.e. the exclusion of cases from food handling.
(b) Bacteriological examination to establish clearance from infection of recovered cases is not necessary.
(c) No action is needed for contacts.
(d) Bacteriological screening of asymptomatic contacts is not indicated except for epidemiological purposes.
(e) Recovered cases with normal stools need not be excluded from their normal activities.

Most of the public health measures appropriate to the control of campylobacter infection apply equally to the control of other microbial infections which are derived from environmental and food sources. These include the provision of safe water and milk supplies; good hygienic practice in animal husbandry and in the handling of raw foods; adequate cooking; kitchen hygiene; and public awareness of the hazard.

(The editors would like to thank Dr Roger Feldman for some of the observations incorporated in this report.)

CASE CONTROL AND OUTBREAK STUDIES

The studies presented confirmed the 2-5 day incubation period and the high attack rates characteristic of milk- and water-borne infection.

Questionnaire analyses established that infection occurred with abdominal pain in the absence of diarrhoea.

Antibody studies to estimate infection rates indicated that 15–20% of the population which was at risk suffered subclinical infection when low test systems were used to measure antibody production.

GENERAL SURVEYS

In the large number of reports of the isolation of thermophilic campylobacters from persons with enteritis, it is generally noted that most isolations are made from infants and small children. This may simply reflect the greater likelihood that diarrhoea in this age group will be reported and investigated. However, those authors who indicate the age-specific attack rates and relate these to the population at risk also suggest that campylobacter enteritis is primarily a disease of the very young. The situation is perhaps analogous to poliomyelitis before the introduction of vaccination where, in areas of high endemicity, children were infected early in life; in developed countries, however, contact with the virus was likely to be delayed.

In several reports isolation rates of **C. jejuni** are compared with those of other enteric pathogens. It is commonly observed that campylobacter is the pathogen most frequently isolated, the rate depending on the age of the population sampled, the relative sensitivity of the techniques and the prevalence of other pathogens in the area. Several authors describe the detection of campylobacters in association with other pathogenic bacteria or viruses.

Those who investigated asymptomatic contacts of cases of **C. jejuni** report isolation rates three or four times higher than those from randomly selected healthy people. This is generally the result of exposure to a common source rather than person to person spread.

ANIMAL AND ENVIRONMENTAL SOURCES

Reports from many surveys of farm animals and poultry demonstrate high carriage rates of thermophilic campylobacters, especially in chickens and pigs. It is suggested that chicken is likely to pose a greater hazard to the consumer than pork because of the greater opportunities for cross-contamination and survival of the organism in chicken processing plants compared with slaughterhouses (see also report of informal meeting on pp. 175–176).

Wild birds and game animals have also been shown to carry campylobacters, reflecting the problem of environmental contamination and the routes of infection to domestic animals and man.

Infection in cattle has been studied and serotypes of **C. jejuni** which are common in human infection have been shown to persist in beef and dairy herds.

SURVIVAL EXPERIMENTS

Since thermophilic campylobacters are unlikely to encounter environmental conditions in which they can multiply, work has been directed to elucidating the factors which favour survival. These include low temperature and pH above 6.

In water, survival is reduced in chlorinated water compared with unchlorinated or polluted water. In milk, survival is prolonged and is only reduced when the pH falls by souring of raw milk. In meats the organisms survive for several days and survival is not appreciably influenced by competitive flora.

Surfaces in kitchens and factories are readily contaminated by raw poultry and campylobacters can survive in moist conditions, emphasising the need for adequate and frequent cleaning.

A. D. Pearson

Public Health Laboratory,
Southampton, UK

J. R. Davies

Public Health Laboratory Service Headquarters,
London, UK

Abstracts of Papers Presented

A. EPIDEMIOLOGY

1. Case control studies

The transmission of *Campylobacter jejuni* infection in a case control study

M. Santosham, E. Walter, L. Magder, V. Sehgal, T. Ireland, W. Spira and R. Black

The Johns Hopkins University, Infectious Enteric Disease Study Center, PO Box 1240, Whiteriver, Arizona 85941, USA

A case control study was conducted to determine possible risk factors and vehicles of transmission of **Campylobacter jejuni**. Index cases were selected from patients seen at the US Public Health Hospital at Whiteriver, Arizona, USA, with confirmed **C. jejuni**-associated diarrhea. Age- and sex-matched controls were selected from the house closest to that of the index case in which no one reported having diarrhea. Households were visited 2-6 days after the index case came to the clinic. Members were questioned about the occurrence of diarrheal illness, food and water consumed in the previous week, sanitary facilities and presence of animals in the house. Rectal swabs were obtained from consenting individuals and from animals.

Twenty household pairs were studied. Nine of 20 index cases were male; 13 of 20 were less than 3 years old and 16 of 20 were less than 6 years old. The only significant difference between case and control households was that 12 of 72 (17%) case family contacts were infected compared to none of 57 contacts in control families ($P < 0.01$). The rate of infection in contacts was significantly associated with age: less than 6 years, nine of 27 (33%) positive; 6-14 years, two of 28 (11%) positive; 15 years and over, one of 27 (4%) positive ($P < 0.01$). Animals harboring **C. jejuni** were detected in only four of 20 case households compared with two of 20 control households. There were no statistically significant differences in the other factors examined. These results suggest that, in this environment, **C. jejuni** may be transmitted to children, primarily by siblings, in the household rather than by animal contacts.

Campylobacter enteritis in an industrial country: epidemiologic features in urban and rural areas

M. Kist

Centre for Hygiene, University of Freiburg, Hermann-Herder-Strasse 11, 7800 Freiburg, Federal Republic of Germany

Over a two-year period stool specimens from 6806 enteritis patients were investigated for **Campylobacter jejuni/coli**. Some 3726 patients came from urban and 3080 from rural areas; 51% were male and 49% female. The number of outpatients was higher in the rural population (55%) compared with the urban population (44%). Clinical and epidemiological data were obtained by questionnaire and compared with data from sex- and age-matched healthy control groups. Campylobacters were isolated from 306 (4.5%) of the enteritis patients. The isolation rate was higher in rural areas (6%) than urban areas (3.2%), and was most frequent in rural outpatients (9%). The highest age-dependent isolation rates were found in the 5–9 year old male outpatient group: here campylobacters were isolated from 13.3% of urban patients and 17.5% of rural patients.

Significantly more male patients (65%) were infected with campylobacter than female patients (35%). This was, however, predominantly due to the in-patients, especially to the 20–60 year age group. Sex distribution was not significantly different when rural patients were compared with urban ones. Therefore one can conclude that the higher isolation rate in male patients is due to more severe disease rather than epidemiological reasons, suggesting a possible hormone-dependent phenomenon.

Interesting differences in epidemiological features were found in both groups. Broiler chickens seem to play a more important role in urban patients ($P < 0.01$), whereas raw milk was an important infection source only in rural areas ($P < 0.001$). Interestingly enough no differences were found concerning the role of household and farm animals, which were not found to be significant sources of infections. The overall frequency of infection in contact persons did not differ markedly between patients from rural and urban areas ($P < 0.05$); it was highest in young boys (55%) and adult females (52%), suggesting a human-to-human spread of the infection from mother to child. The higher frequency of campylobacter infections in rural areas can probably be explained by epidemiological factors, especially different diet habits.

Epidemiological investigations on Campylobacter in households with a primary infection

J. Oosterom,* C. H. den Uyl,* J. R. J. Banffer† and J. Huisman†

*National Institute of Public Health, Laboratory for Zoonoses and Food Microbiology, PO Box 1, 3720 BA Bilthoven, The Netherlands, and †Municipal Public Health Service, PO Box 333, 3000 AH Rotterdam, The Netherlands

Fifty-four households living in the region of Rotterdam in which a primary infection with **Campylobacter jejuni** occurred were investigated. An enquiry was made regarding clinical features, use of medicines, enteritis in household members, foods eaten before onset of disease, the presence of pet animals, etc. Data from each household were compared with those of a control household living in the same street. Bacteriological and serological investigations were carried out in the index households. For the serological examination an ELISA system, in which disintegrated whole cells were used as antigen, was used.

The most important findings from these investigations were as follows:

(1) The consumption of poultry meat was a highly significant factor for the acquisition of campylobacter enteritis. Other foods, including pork, beef, mutton and milk, were not significantly associated.

(2) Another significant factor was eating at a barbecue, which in all instances was associated with the consumption of chicken meat. Other methods of food preparation, including eating at restaurants, were not significant.

(3) The use of erythromycin had no influence on the duration of the disease; it only shortened the excretion period.

(4) Campylobacters were isolated from only 0.5% of swabs from kitchens. In an earlier study 18% of swabs from kitchens were positive for salmonellae.

(5) An ELISA system is a suitable tool for the detection of campylobacter antibodies.

Family studies of Campylobacter jejuni in Bangladesh: implications for pathogenesis and transmission

R. I. Glass, B. J. Stoll, M. I. Huq, M. Struelens and A. K. M. G. Kibriya

International Centre for Diarrhoeal Disease Research - Bangladesh, GPO Box 128, Dhaka-2, Bangladesh, and The Centers for Disease Control, Atlanta, Georgia, USA

Family members of diarrhoeal patients with campylobacters and control patients (with diarrhoea from whom campylobacters were not isolated) who were treated at the Dhaka Hospital of the ICCDR-B, were followed for 2 or more weeks to determine their pattern of infection, disease, and serologic response. Campylobacters isolated from patients, their household contacts and household animals were serotyped to study transmission from animals to man and to determine if prolonged excretion of campylobacters seen in some individuals was of a single serotype.

On the first home visit, campylobacters were isolated from 9% of 314 contacts of cases versus 2% of 267 controls ($P < 0.01$). Campylobacters were more likely to be isolated from contacts than controls (21% versus 13%; $P < 0.01$) at least once during a 2 week follow-up period of alternate day visits. The median duration of excretion of campylobacters was 8 days in contacts who developed diarrhoea versus 1.5 days in contacts with asymptomatic infections. Infants and young children were more frequently infected. The disease-to-infection rate decreased continuously with increasing age from 78% for infants less than 1 year to 21% in children of

5-14 years. More index patients with diarrhoea had elevated convalescent titres (of more than 1:20) by complement fixation than their matched controls (16 of 47 versus two of 48; P < 0.01).

Preliminary transmission data indicate that 25% of domestic chickens are infected with campylobacters, yet families with a member infected with campylobacters were no more likely to have chickens at home than families with no one infected. Other results of serotyping and serologic response will be reviewed. These studies suggest that campylobacters are pathogenic in Bangladesh, particularly among infants and small children. Development of immunity early in life could explain the decreased disease-to-infection rate with increasing age. Immunity would also explain the high rate of asymptomatic infection, the lack of a distinct clinical presentation, and the high rate of mixed enteric infection with campylobacters in older children and adults, as previously reported by us from Bangladesh. These latter aspects distinguish the epidemiology of infection with this agent in populations from developed versus developing countries.

2. Outbreak studies

Outbreak of campylobacter enteritis involving over 500 participants in a jogging rally

H. Stalder, R. Isler, W. Stutz, M. Salfinger, S. Lauwers and W. Vischer

Medizinische Klinik, Kantonsspital, 4410 Liestal, Switzerland

We describe an outbreak of enteritis due to **Campylobacter jejuni** in participants in a jogging rally. Over 500 of about 800 runners became ill. **C. jejuni** was the only organism isolated from the 22 participants for whom stool cultures were carried out. By means of a questionnaire, information was obtained about food consumption, incubation period, duration of illness and symptoms. A drink prepared with raw milk was incriminated as the vehicle of the outbreak. Some 510 of 659 milk consumers became ill (attack rate 77.4%). The mean incubation period was 3.2 days and the mean duration of illness 4.4 days. The most common symptoms were: diarrhoea (89%), abdominal cramps (84.7%), fever (62.7%), headache (32.9%) and vomiting (13.1%). Secondary cases were rare. Fourteen isolates from affected persons were serotyped by passive haemagglutination. Thirteen were identified as type 2 whereas one isolate reacted only slightly with type 2 antiserum and therefore remained untypable. This type was otherwise very rarely found in our region. The unpasteurised milk originated from three farms with a total of 44 cows. Of these, seven excreted **C. jejuni** in their faeces. Six of these isolates belonged to the commoner serotypes in our region, whereas one cow excreted the incriminated type 2. We conclude that the milk of a single cow was probably contaminated faecally with **C. jejuni**, and that this was the origin of illness in over 500 persons.

Epidemiology of an outbreak of milk-borne enteritis in a residential school

P. G. Wilson,* J. R. Davies,† T. W. Hoskins,§ K. P. Lander,** H. Lior,†† D. M. Jones§§ and A. D. Pearson***

*Control of Infection Unit, Tower Hill, Bristol, UK; †Public Health Laboratory Service, London, UK; §Christ's Hospital, Horsham, UK; **Central Veterinary Laboratory, Weybridge, UK; ††Laboratory Center for Disease Control, Ottawa, Canada; §§Public Health Laboratory, Manchester, UK; and ***Public Health Laboratory, Southampton, UK

The outbreak began with 29 boys reporting symptoms of diarrhoea, abdominal pain or vomiting to the school medical officer on Tuesday 16 March 1982. The epidemic reached a peak the next day with 67 boys reporting ill. During the week of the outbreak a total of 189 boys were seen by the medical officer and 102 admitted to the school infirmary, almost all of whom were pyrexial. An analysis of the clinical findings in relation to day of onset, serological responses and complications is given by Hoskins and Davies (see abstract on p. 14).

A questionnaire was distributed to all pupils and 20 staff in the school and it was completed by 775 (99%) of boys. A total of 518 (67%) had one or more symptoms, of whom 57% had diarrhoea, 30% pain without diarrhoea, and 13% symptoms other than pain or diarrhoea. Diarrhoea was not associated with food or water, but was correlated with milk drinking ($P < 0.05$) and was more common with increasing consumption. An analysis by age group and amount of milk consumed showed that older boys were less likely to have symptoms in spite of a heavier milk consumption.

Specimen faeces were examined from 41 boys. **Campylobacter jejuni** was isolated from 36 (88%) of them and 33 of these strains were available for analysis; all were considered to be of the same serotype (Lior scheme type 7; Penner scheme (modified) type 13). Serological evidence of infection (ELISA; complement fixation; bactericidal test) was found in 82% of boys who had pain and diarrhoea and 44% of boys without symptoms.

Milk was obtained from a farm in the school grounds. Pasteurising equipment had been installed in 1981. Investigation at the farm showed this equipment to be functioning satisfactorily. However, it was possible to bypass the pasteuriser (the farm supplied raw milk to a large processor) and it is conceivable that the school might inadvertantly have been supplied with raw milk. Campylobacters of various serotypes, including the strain responsible for this outbreak, were isolated from rectal swabs from the cows and from a sample of milk from one animal.

Applications of serotyping, biotyping and bactericidal tests to the investigation of a water-borne outbreak of campylobacter gastroenteritis

A. D. Pearson,* **S. R. Palmer**,† H. Lior§ and D. M. Jones**

*Public Health Laboratory, Southampton, UK; †PHLS Communicable Disease Surveillance Centre, London, UK; §Laboratory Center for Disease Control, Ottawa, Canada; and **Public Health Laboratory, Manchester, UK

An outbreak of gastroenteritis affecting over 234 pupils and 23 staff at a private residential school occurred over 2 months in the spring of 1981. Some 37% (234/625) of pupils and 40% (23/57) of the staff reported illness in a questionaire survey. In staff there was a statistically significant association ($P < 0.01$) between reported illness and consumption of water which came from a cold water storage tank. Attack rates in pupils corresponded closely with the distribution of this water supply to their residential houses.

Campylobacters were isolated from the stools of 17 pupils and staff and from two 5 litre water samples taken from the storage tank on 1 June 1981. Both water isolates and 12 human isolates from 11 patients were serotyped according to the schemes of Penner and Lior and biotyped according to the extended system described by Lior. Sera from staff and pupils were obtained 3-7 weeks after the onset of symptoms and antibody titres to **Campylobacter jejuni/coli** estimated by complement-fixation, ELISA and bactericidal tests.

The 12 human isolates fell into two groups: seven were **C. jejuni** biotype III, Lior serotype 6, Penner serotype 6; and five were **C. jejuni** biotype I, Lior serotype 39, Penner serotype 58. One of the adults excreted both serotypes. Both water isolates were serotype 6, biotype III. The results of bactericidal tests correlated closely with the infecting serotype, although an adult with Penner serotype 6 isolated from faeces had antibodies to Penner serotype 41 as well as Penner serotype 6, and in one patient infected with Penner serotype 58, only Penner serotype 6 bactericidal antibodies were detected.

In those from whom **C. jejuni** isolates were not obtained, 34 had Penner serotype 6 bactericidal antibodies, three of whom also had Penner serotype 58 and three of whom also had Penner serotype 41 antibodies. A further four persons had only Penner 41 antibodies.

In staff, the presence of bactericidal, ELISA and CFT antibodies were not significantly associated with illness, although a trend was evident. The presence of antibody detected by the three methods was significantly associated with consumption of water. In those staff who drank water, 25 of 35 (71%) had either bactericidal antibodies or CFT antibodies (titre of 1:8 or more) and 10 of these (40%) were symptomless.

In summary, serological tests suggested the following: (1) the outbreak was due to three distinct serotypes of **C. jejuni**; (2) concurrent infection with at least two serotypes occurred in at least nine of 74 (12%) of those examined; (3) water from the borehole/tank source was the main vehicle of infection; (4) the asymptomatic infection rate in this prolonged water-borne outbreak was 40%.

Antibody response and isolation of Campylobacter jejuni in an outbreak of food-borne enterocolitis

A. Svedhem and H. Gunnarsson

Department of Clinical Bacteriology, Institute of Medical Microbiology, University of Goteborg, Goteborg, Sweden

A hospital staff party was arranged for 106 people. The menu - coq au vin, boiled rice and fresh salad - was prepared in a restaurant kitchen and delivered in canisters. Thirty-two people became ill 1-7 days after the party. Of the 106 participants, 86 were identified, interviewed and examined by stool cultures 10 days after the party. **Campylobacter jejuni** was isolated from 17 people (20%), of whom two were symptomless.

Serum samples were obtained from 82 participants and of these 58 (67%) developed significantly raised levels of IgM and/or IgG antibodies to **C. jejuni** as monitored by DIG-ELISA (diffusion in gel). **C. jejuni** antibodies were detected in 24 of 29 tested serum samples from 32 people with overt symptoms.

The restaurant staff, equipment and the food (except for the salad) were examined for **C. jejuni** with negative results. The most probable reason for this outbreak was a failure of kitchen routine. The raw chickens and the salad were prepared on the same cutting-board in the order mentioned. Raw chickens are usually contaminated with **C. jejuni**.

This outbreak shows the value of diagnostic serology. Compared with stool cultures, the diagnostic rate was raised to around 50% in people with symptoms. Furthermore, over 50% of the participants who remained healthy were shown to have started an active immunological response.

Investigations on Campylobacter spp. in the German Democratic Republic

H. Mochmann and U. Richter

Institut fur Infektionskrankheiten im Kindesalter im Stadtischen Klinikum Berlin-Buch, Wiltbergstrasse 50, 1115 Berlin, German Democratic Republic

Since April 1982 we have examined stool specimens from patients suffering from diarrhoea for campylobacters.

First, we found these organisms in an outbreak of enteritis in a boarding school in Berlin. A total of 197 children and pupils between 9 and 20 years old fell ill with fever, diarrhoea and abdominal cramps. Out of 39 stool specimens from these patients, we isolated 15 strains of **Campylobacter jejuni**. Other enteropathogenic bacteria and rotaviruses were not detected. Because this outbreak had an explosive course, we presume that the source of infection was food.

Since that time we have regularly isolated these organisms from sporadic enteritic cases. Out of 4478 stool specimens from enteric cases, 195 (4.3%) were positive. Out of 1878 stool specimens from healthy persons, seven (0.4%) were positive. Tentative investigations of animal material showed that faecal campylobacters occur in poultry, pigs and calves in our country.

Incidents of campylobacter enteritis in Japan

R. Sakazaki, K. Tamura and S. Kuramochi

National Institute of Health, Kamiosaki, Shinagawa-ku, Tokyo, Japan

The working group on diarrhoeal disease supported by the Ministry of Health, Japan, has conducted a survey of campylobacter enteritis since 1978. During the years 1979-83, 83 outbreaks of campylobacter infection were reported, although the incidents were less frequent than those of infections with **Vibrio parahaemolyticus** and salmonellae. Most of the incidents were at elementary schools. Since most elementary schools in Japan provide a midday meal, it is probable that school meals played an important part in these outbreaks. Despite much effort, however, sources of infection were not established in most of the incidents. An epidemic of diarrhoeal disease involving 7000 persons occurred at a superstore in 1982. In this epidemic campylobacters were found in patients together with enterotoxigenic **Escherichia coli**, and water-borne infection was suggested.

In contrast to general outbreaks, campylobacters were responsible for the largest proportion of sporadic cases of gastroenteritis; the organism was isolated from an average of 66% of outpatients with bacterial diarrhoea in large hospitals and from 40-45% of children suffering from gastroenteritis in practitioner's offices. Isolation of campylobacters from sporadic cases was highest in May to September; it decreased in the cold season.

Occurrence and significance of Campylobacter jejuni in Yamaguchi, Japan

S. Matsusaki and A. Katayama

Yamaguchi Prefectural Research Institute of Health, 5-67 2-chome, Aoi, Yamaguchi City, Japan

Seven outbreaks of food poisoning due to **Campylobacter jejuni/coli** involving a total of 1324 patients have been recorded in Yamaguchi since 1980, and the number accounted for 14.9% of all cases of outbreaks reported during the same period. In sporadic cases, **C. jejuni/coli** was isolated from 98 (39.4%) of 247 stool samples of children with acute enteritis. Fifty-eight (1.36%) of 4188 faecal specimens of healthy people aged 2-84 years were also culture-positive, and children under 10 years old showed the highest isolation rate (2.92%).

The organism was detected in wild birds (57 of 340), wild mammals (two of 21), cows (six of 57), pigs (137 of 195), dogs (12 of 186), cats (seven of 29), live chickens (179 of 199) and dressed chickens in markets (59 of 114), but in none of 293 foodstuffs, 57 cold-blooded animals or 12 samples of river water. In the case of wild birds, the frequency of isolation among different species was varied; for example, crows had a high rate of isolation (23 of 40) but pheasants had a low one (none of 30).

It is clear the **C. jejuni/coli** is widely carried in domestic and wild animals, and so food and other environmental sources may be contaminated with this organism. In fact, we confirmed that chicken meats were contaminated with **C. jejuni/coli** during processing at poultry plants. This organism was isolated from swab samples from working equipment (42 of 104), eviscerated chickens (26 of 55) and chicken meat (20 of 30).

Distribution of **C. jejuni** and **C. coli** in various specimens was examined. All strains from pigs and many from wild birds were identified as **C. coli**, whereas most of the strains from other specimens were **C. jejuni**.

Outbreak of water-borne enteritis in a kindergarten

V. Brckovic, A. Kalenic and **I. Vodopija**

Zagreb Institute of Public Health, 41000 Zagreb, Mirogojska 16, Yugoslavia

An outbreak of acute diarrhoeal infection appeared in a kindergarten in Zagreb in June 1983. Among 224 exposed persons the symptoms of enteritis were diagnosed in 122 persons. The course of the outbreak showed a sudden increase 2 days after the beginning of the outbreak. In a period of 1 week (6–11 June), 77 out of a total of 122 became ill. Afterwards the outbreak slowly subsided, with the tail of the outbreak appearing from 20 to 22 June and involving eight persons.

Stool specimens were examined from 167 persons (110 diseased and 57 healthy). Agents of enteritis were isolated from 74 diseased and two healthy persons, as follows: **Shigella sonnei** in 52 persons, **Campylobacter jejuni/coli** in 32 and **Giardia lamblia** in 16 persons. Multiple isolation of agents is presented in the following table:

Agent	No. of patients
Sh. sonnei	29
Sh. sonnei + C. jejuni/coli	15
Sh. sonnei + G. lamblia	8
C. jejuni/coli	16
G. lamblia	6
Total	74

All patients were treated with sulphometoxasol + trimethoprim and metronidazole for a period of 5 days.

Out of 32 **C. jejuni/coli** strains, nine were biotyped; seven were found to be **C. coli** and two **C. jejuni** biotype 1.

The available data and test results suggest that the well water supplying the kindergarten might have been contaminated. Agents of enteritis were not determined in the water samples but **Sh. sonnei** phages were found.

3. General Surveys

Observations regarding 202 campylobacter enteritis outbreaks in northern Israel from July 1979 to February 1983

M. Shmilovitz and B. Kretzer

W. Hirsch Regional Microbiology Laboratory, Kupat Holim, Haifa and Western Galilee, Israel

Of 3939 **Campylobacter jejuni** enteritis patients, detected during a period of 43 months, 872 (22.1%) were involved in 202 outbreaks. Two-thirds (134) of the 202 outbreaks, comprising 733 or 84.1% of the patients, occurred in institutions, whereas the remaining third, comprising 139 or 15.9% of the patients, appeared in families.

Distribution of the outbreaks by area of location showed that all but two of the 134 institutional outbreaks occurred in rural areas, all collective settlements (kibbutzim), in contrast to only seven of the 68 family outbreaks.

Some 95.6% of the family outbreaks comprised two cases, whereas the same figure in institutions was only 31.3%. On the other hand, no more than three cases were noted in family outbreaks, whereas in half of the institutional outbreaks there were between four and 34 patients per outbreak. Although the outbreaks were generally small, ranging from two to 34 patients, a marked difference was seen between family and institutional outbreaks. Thus, the average number of cases was 5.47 per institutional outbreak versus only 2.04 per family outbreak. This observation may be correlated with the peculiarity of the institutional outbreaks, which generally were in collective settlements (kibbutzim) located in rural areas with a large animal population in the environment.

Distribution of the patients by age group showed that the percentage of cases under the age of 5 years was not significantly different (10–19%) between institutional and family outbreaks, whereas with cases over 5 years old a very striking difference (66–161%) was noted.

The seasonal distribution of the outbreaks indicate that from 1980 to 1982 the peak incidence, namely 48.9% of all outbreaks, occurred during the months April–July. Thus, the occurrence of nearly a half of the outbreaks during these months appeared to be different from other enteric bacterial infections, mainly due to shigellae, the prevalent bacterial agent of diarrhoeal diseases in Israel, where the most frequent outbreaks occurred during July–September.

In 29 of 67 kibbutzim (43.3%) outbreaks occurred again, between two and seven times at intervals of 2–29 months. The repeated outbreaks in over two-fifths of the affected collective settlements suggested an endemic characteristic of **C. jejuni** infections. Nevertheless, more observations in this respect, supported by typing of the isolates, are needed.

In two institutional outbreaks there were six asymptomatic but bacteriologically positive cases. Evidence of a significant and dynamic titre of agglutinins toward the homologous isolates enabled these cases to be differentiated from healthy carriers. Conversely, some three symptomatic but bacteriologically negative cases were confirmed by the presence of a significant titre of agglutinins toward the outbreak strain.

Fifty-three of the outbreaks were screened with polyvalent and monovalent antisera provided by the Campylobacter Centre in Jerusalem. In 25 of these (47.2%), the isolates from the same outbreak gave different patterns, indicating infection with more than one strain. Such a proportion of outbreaks with multiple strains was very rarely encountered in our large experience with other enteric bacterial infections, such as with shigellae or with salmonellae.

Campylobacter infection in Scotland, 1978–82

J. C. M. Sharp

Communicable Diseases (Scotland) Unit, Ruchill Hospital, Glasgow G20 9NB, UK

The component countries of the UK share many demographic and other features, yet differences occur in the epidemiology of campylobacter infections. The seasonal distribution in Scotland does not feature the predominance in the third quarter apparent in England and Wales, and there is a striking preponderence of pre-school children. The male excess in children of all ages contrasts with an excess of females in young adults. During 1978-82, 7808 campylobacter infections (annual attack rate of 31.0 per 100,000) were reported, with less than 4% imported from overseas.

Poultry, red meats and seafood were implicated in small-scale outbreaks. Raw milk caused seven outbreaks affecting 926 persons (range two to 648), and it was a suspected source in numerous sporadic cases. The introduction of compulsory heat treatment of milk in Scotland in August 1983 will provide a unique opportunity to study its effect on disease incidence. Campylobacter isolates from animals included dogs (33), cattle (22), pigs (seven), sheep (five), cats (five) and poultry (five) and food samples such as poultry meat, pork, milk, and walnut cheese. Surveys of seagulls also revealed many isolations.

In 1980, Scotland became the first country to participate in a WHO Surveillance Programme of Foodborne Infections in Europe, in consequence of which more meaningful data on human campylobacter infections are emerging.

Epidemiological differences in campylobacter infections in urban and rural communities in Scotland

C. J. Sibbald

Environmental Health Department, Public Health Chambers, Johnston Terrace, Edinburgh EH1 2PP, UK

Investigation of 1848 patients with campylobacter infection within the city of Edinburgh over a 5 year period (annual attack rate 81.2 per 100,000) revealed certain trends in relation to attack rates in various age groups.

As there is a very low sale of unpasteurised milk in Edinburgh (the food vehicle most frequently incriminated elsewhere in Britain), it was considered unlikely that this was responsible for many infections. Accordingly, a study was undertaken to compare the data for Edinburgh from 1978 to 1982 with the national picture in Scotland and also various regions within the country. In general, urban areas in Scotland have similar age case incidence distributions, with peaks occurring in children and younger adults. Rural areas showed different distributions when compared with urban areas. Possible reasons for this are being examined, including the availability of unpasteurised milk and the possibility of acquired immunity to campylobacter enteritis after repeated dosing with low numbers of the organism.

Epidemiological survey of campylobacter infections in children in the south-west of France

F. Megraud, Z. Elharrif and J. Latrille

Departement de Bacteriologie, Hopital des Enfants, Bordeaux, France

Over a period of 3 years and 9 months (July 1979–March 1983), we looked for thermophilic campylobacters by plating, on Butzler's medium, faeces from children with intestinal symptoms referred to our hospital. This children's hospital is the only one for a population of about 700,000 inhabitants. We found 207 campylobacters (2.6%) among 7912 stools tested, compared with 393 salmonellae (4.9%), 92 shigellae (1.1%) and 36 **Yersinia enterocolitica** (0.4%). We reviewed 184 case histories.

The distribution according to age showed the highest incidence during infancy: 47% before 1 year including six cases in newborns, 22% between 1 and 2 years, 18% between 2 and 5 years, and 12% between 5 and 15 years. No seasonal pattern was noted. Some 25% of the children were from an immigrant population, mainly from North Africa. In addition to campylobacters, 20% of the children had another enteropathogenic microorganism in the stools and 17% had another infectious disease; 93% were hospitalised. The source of infection was unknown in most of the cases. Some 8% were infected abroad. Most of the cases were sporadic: only 12 out of 184 had a history of a family outbreak. We noticed that one case of diarrhoea occurred after the death of a pet guinea-pig, itself a victim of diarrhoea. A survey of campylobacters in animal faeces from a local slaughterhouse showed similar incidences in our region as in others: pigs (88%), chickens (76%), cows (36%) and sheep (26%).

These data confirm the importance of campylobacter infections in infants in a temperate area.

Campylobacter enteritis: incidence in a general hospital in Madrid during a five-year period

M. Lopez-Brea, J. Gonzalez Sainz and M. Baquero

Department of Microbiology, Centro Ramon y Cajal, Madrid 23, Spain

Campylobacter enteritis is a worldwide infection and apparently an important cause of enteritis, particularly in children. The first identification in Spain occurred in 1978 [1]. During a five year period (1978–82), we cultured 7833 stool specimens from children and adults (in-patients and out-patients) at the Centro Ramon y Cajal, Madrid. Faeces were cultured on horse blood agar containing vancomycin (10 mg/l), polymyxin B (2500 i.u./l) and trimethoprim (5 mg/l). Plates were incubated overnight at 43 °C in a jar (without catalyst) containing an activated Gas-Pak under partial vacuum (500 mmHg).

Campylobacters were cultured from 106 (1.35%) of the 7833 faeces specimens examined; the 106 specimens represented 93 patients with diarrhoea. The highest isolation rate was in children less than 1 year old (35 of 93).

Sera from 49 children without gastrointestinal symptoms (aged 2–13 years, mean 8.2 years) were tested for complement fixing antibody to an antigen consisting of a sonicate of six campylobacter strains of different serotypes. Eighteen (37%) were positive at a titre of 1:2 or more.

Our results show that campylobacter enteritis affects people of all ages, but with a predominance in young children. Children without gastrointestinal symptoms may have complement fixing antibodies to campylobacter.

REFERENCE

1. M. Lopez-Brea, D. Molina and M. Baquero. Campylobacter in Spain. Transactions of the Royal Society of Tropical Medicine and Hygiene, 1979, **73**, 474.

Human campylobacteriosis in Ferrara (Italy): incidence and characteristics of isolates

P. Maini, I. Piva and G. Bucci

Presidio Multizonale di Preventione, C. so Giovecca 169, 44100 Ferrara, Italy

In 1982, stool specimens from 969 subjects were submitted to our Public Health Laboratory for bacterial culture. About one in five were for screening normal people. Some 70% were children under 12 years old, of whom 88 were admitted to hospital on account of enteritis. Specimens were cultured for salmonellae, shigellae, yersiniae, **Campylobacter jejuni/coli** and **Vibrio parahaemolyticus** (summer months). Selected specimens (291) were tested for rotavirus. The isolation rates were as follows: salmonellae 8.4%, campylobacters 4.1%, yersiniae 1.4%, shigellae and vibrios 0%; rotavirus 11.3%. The ratio of hospitalised to non-hospitalised positive children was: salmonellae 0.43:1, rotavirus 0.30:1, campylobacters 0.08:1. Of hospitalised children, 25% had salmonellae, 26% rotavirus, but none had yersiniae.

Of 40 subjects positive for campylobacters, 37 were children, 29 of them under 3 years of age (three were admitted to hospital). Four non-hospitalised children had, besides campylobacters, other pathogens: one rotavirus, one yersinia, two salmonellae (this can pose problems for therapy). Campylobacter isolations were more frequent in warm months, with a peak of 10.4% in September. However, in January, we had a small outbreak of campylobacter enteritis in a nursery. Nursery staff were not involved (cultures and serology negative).

All cases of campylobacter enteritis had an uncomplicated course. Bloody stools, profuse diarrhoea and high fever were rarely present. Campylobacters were found in two children and one adult who were apparently symptomless.

Biotyping was performed according to Skirrow: one strain was not inhibited by nalidixic acid, yet it was hippurate positive.

Serotyping (performed by Dr S. Lauwers, Brussels) showed that the commonest serotypes were 2 and 1.

Susceptibility to nine antimicrobial drugs was tested: no resistance to erythromycin was found.

Twenty-one single and four paired sera from patients were tested by tube agglutination with homologous strains and by complement fixation with a commercial antigen. Both methods gave substantially concordant results.

Campylobacteriosis in the Gorizia and Rovigo area: a new problem of public health

G. Benzi,* **D. Crotti†** and P. Pugina*

*Ospedale Civile Rovigo, Servizio Microbiologia, via Tre Martiri, 45100 Rovigo, and †Ospedale Civile Gorizia, Servizio Microbiologia, 34170 Gorizia, Italy

From 1 October 1982 to 28 February 1983 we analysed 2203 samples of stools from people living in the areas surrounding Rovigo and Gorizia. We isolated 31 strains (1.4%) of **Campylobacter jejuni** and **C. coli**; 28 strains (5.6%) were isolated from patients with gastroenteritis (496), and three strains (0.2%) from healthy people (1707). Of the 31 strains isolated, 26 (84%) were **C. jejuni**, and four (13%) **C. coli**.

From the same group of people, and in the same period, we isolated 84 salmonellas (3.8%); 23 strains (1.3%) were from healthy people, and 61 strains (12.3%) from people with gastroenteritis. From the same group, **Yersinia enterocolotica** was isolated eight times (0.4%); two strains (0.4%) were from patients with gastroenteritis, and six strains (0.4%) from healthy people.

We also looked for the presence of anti-campylobacter antibodies among the inhabitants of our area. Some 218 ill and healthy people were examined. We commonly found specific antibodies in healthy people, which indicates a higher prevalence of the microorganism than found by direct bacteriological methods. We isolated 90 strains (19%) of **C. jejuni** and **C. coli** from 475 stool samples from birds (poultry, crows, seagulls, pheasants, doves) and mammals (dogs, oxen, pigs).

Campylobacter enteritis in Hungary – experiences of a three-year study in Pest county

M. M. Adam

National Institute of Hygiene, 2-6 Gyali ut, Budapest IX, Hungary H-1966

In the years 1980-2 the culturing of campylobacters was successively started in 13 laboratories of the Hungarian Public Health Service. Faecal samples from 5880 (1980), 31,778 (1981) and 63,837 (1982) patients with enteritis were tested. Campylobacters were isolated from 9.2, 6.1 and 4.0% of samples respectively. Out of a total of 11,881 asymptomatic contacts of different ages the isolation rate was 3.1%, and out of 4195 healthy people it was 1.7%. In Pest county the annual incidences of campylobacter enteritis were 6.8, 6.0 and 2.0% in 3403, 5942 and 6265 patients respectively, whereas the incidences of salmonellosis were 3.1, 2.5 and 3.8% and those of shigellosis 0.6, 0.2 and 0.2%. Campylobacter enteritis was most frequent in October 1980 (8.6%), in February 1981 (11.4%), in May 1981 (10.2%), and in May and December 1982 (both 3.3%). The highest incidences were in infants (9.7, 13.8 and 4.3%) and in children aged 1–5 years (10.1, 7.8 and 3.0%). Except for infants of 1–5 years of age in 1981, males were more frequently affected by campylobacter enteritis. Watery and slimy diarrhoea occurred in 41.6%, bloody diarrhoea in 25.9%, vomiting in 4.0%, abdominal pain in 25.2%, and pyrexia in 35.7%. The illness was mild in 13.4%, severe in 3.1% and lasted on average 7.3 days. Some 80–91% of isolates were sensitive to tetracycline and 13–39% were sensitive to ampicillin. Resistance to erythromycin and nalidixic acid was rare.

Epidemiology of campylobacters in Zagreb, Yugoslavia

S. Kalenic,* M. B. Skirrow,† B. Gmajnicki,* Z. Baklaic* and **I. Vodopija***

*Zagreb Institute of Public Health, 41000 Zagreb, Mirogojska 16, Yugoslavia, and †Worcester Royal Infirmary, Worcester WR1 3AS, UK

Campylobacter jejuni/coli is an important cause of diarrhoeal disease in Zagreb. In 1982 the number of **C. jejuni/coli** isolates outnumbered all other bacterial causes of diarrhoeal disease: it was isolated in 679 patients, compared to 636 isolates of shigellae, 481 of salmonellae and 32 of yersiniae in a total of 5316 patients with enteritis.

BIOTYPE DISTRIBUTION OF CAMPYLOBACTER JEJUNI/COLI In a 12 month period (September 1982–August 1983) 280 **C. jejuni/coli** strains were biotyped; 56.1% were **C. coli**, 41.1% were **C. jejuni** biotype 1, 2.5% were **C. jejuni** biotype 2, and 0.3% were hippurate negative atypical group.

There was a striking difference in the seasonal distribution of **C. jejuni** and **C. coli**: in the spring (March) **C. jejuni** accounted for nearly 90% of isolates, whereas in autumn (September–November) almost all isolates were **C. coli**. The extraordinary preponderance of **C. coli** (to the best of our knowledge not reported from anywhere else) might be explained by the popularity of home rearing of pigs in the Zagreb region. It is an almost universal practice for rural families to rear four or five pigs for home slaughter in the autumn and sale to townsfolk, as well as for their own consumption. Spit-roast piglets (12–15 kg) are particularly popular.

AGE DEPENDENCE OF CAMPYLOBACTER JEJUNI/COLI CARRIAGE Age distribution of persons with **C. jejuni/coli** shows that in the first year of life 49.6% of all enteritis cases are caused by **C. jejuni/coli**, whereas in the second year of life this frequency is reduced to 24.9%, falling sharply in the third year to 7.3% and remaining at that level (between 1.9 and 9.6%) for the other age groups. The high percentage of infections in infancy and early childhood defines **C. jejuni/coli** diarrhoea as an infection of first contact. On the other hand, **C. jejuni/coli** in healthy people is noticeable only above the age of 5 years (1% in the age group 5–9 years;

subsequently 2–3% for all other groups up to 59). Healthy contacts in households of campylobacter enteritis patients constitute a separate group with a **C. jejuni/coli** isolation rate of 12.7%.

Campylobacter enteritis in Tokyo, April 1979–March 1983: epidemiological and clinical studies

M. Murata, T. Fukami and Y. Imagawa

Department of Infectious Diseases, Tokyo Metropolitan Bokutoh Hospital, 4-23-15 Kotobashi, Sumida-ku, Tokyo, Japan

Campylobacter enteritis has been studied in Bokutoh Hospital since April 1979. In Tokyo **Campylobacter jejuni** is the most common pathogen in children suspected of having bacterial enteritis. Its isolation rate has increased recently to 18%. This figure was more than three times that of **Salmonella** spp. In an age distribution study, most isolations were from 2 year old children, but the age-specific isolation rate was highest in patients aged 5–14 years (24.2%). The seasonal variation of **C. jejuni** infection was not as remarkable as that of **Salmonella** spp., but a considerable increase was noticed in June and July of 1981 and 1982. The subjects of this study were 318 children in outpatient clinics and 24 hospitalised children. Their clinical features were similar to those already reported, but there were some clinical differences between age groups. Bloody stools were more frequent (50%) and fever was less frequent (40%) in young infants than in children of school age (bloody stool 20%, fever 80%). Eight patients had two episodes of campylobacter enteritis at intervals of 2 months to 3 years. The serotypes of the strains which were isolated from the two episodes were examined in four patients. Three patients had different serotypes of **C. jejuni** and one had untypable serotypes of **C. coli**.

A study of campylobacter enteritis in Bombay

R. B. Pal and C. K. Deshpande

Department of Microbiology, Seth G.S. Medical College, Parel, Bombay 400 012, India

In a study of 1280 cases of diarrhoea, the incidence of campylobacter enteritis was found to be 8.6%. Patients of all age groups were affected, but children under 10 years old accounted for 77% of cases. Blood and mucus in stools was noticed in 100% and 80.9% of cases respectively. About 71% of patients were febrile and about 66% of cases had abdominal pain, which was periumbilical. Organisms were isolated from the blood of 10.6% of febrile cases. All the strains were found to be sensitive to chloramphenicol, furazolidone, gentamicin, kanamycin, metronidazole and neomycin. All the strains were resistant to penicillin and sulphadiazine. Resistance to erythromycin and tetracycline was found in 5.5% and 3.7% of strains.

An isolation rate of 4.3% was obtained in 258 normal controls. Vegetables (330), egg shells (280), fishes (150) and fowl intestinal contents were studied for the vehicle and source of human infection. **Campylobacter jejuni** was isolated from 8.9% and 60% of egg shells and intestinal contents of fowls respectively. Samples of vegetables and fishes were negative for **C. jejuni**. Strong evidence of transmission from person to person was found. Cattle, fowls and pet animals are among the suspected sources of infection. Paired sera examined by passive haemagglutination against the patient's own strain showed fourfold or higher rises in antibody titre in 47% of cases. Pathogenicity was tested in rabbits, dogs, fowls and infant mice. Enterotoxins were not detected, but an invasive ability of organisms was noticed in dogs and fowls.

Clinical, bacteriological and environmental studies on Campylobacter jejuni in Calcutta, India

G. Balakrish Nair, S. Chowdhury, S. K. Bhattacharya and S. C. Pal

National Institute of Cholera and Enteric Diseases, P-33, CIT Scheme XM, Beliaghata, Calcutta 700 010, India

In a study spanning a period of 16 months, **Campylobacter jejuni** was isolated from 20 (6.7%) of 297 patients suffering from acute diarrhoea and from two (3.6%) of 56 asymptomatic healthy people. In 12 patients, **C. jejuni** was found in association with **Vibrio cholerae** biotype El Tor (Ogawa); it was the sole bacterial pathogen in only seven cases. No age- or sex-specific incidence was observed, nor was any kind of seasonal variation discernible during the period of investigation. Review of the 20 cases excreting **C. jejuni** revealed no distinct clinical presentation. Both the dysenteric and diarrhoeal syndromes were encountered, the latter being predominant. Additionally, 63% of chicken intestinal samples obtained from a poultry market harboured **C. jejuni**. No clear-cut biotypic difference could be identified among the human and chicken isolates, and all isolates were sensitive to the most commonly used antibiotics.

Isolation of Campylobacter jejuni in Lagos, Nigeria. A "new" bacterial agent of diarrhoea

A. O. Coker and O. Dosunmu-Ogunbi

Department of Microbiology and Parasitology, Lagos University Teaching Hospital, PMB 12003, Lagos, Nigeria

Some 436 stool specimens submitted to the Department of Microbiology and Parasitology of the Lagos University Teaching Hospital and Gbaja Health Centre between August 1981 and March 1982 were processed for **Campylobacter jejuni**. Twelve strains of **C. jejuni** were isolated and confirmed. Stool specimens were streaked on Skirrow's and Butzler's type media. We had to discontinue with the Skirrow's medium because horse blood, which is an important ingredient, is very difficult to obtain in Lagos. Plates were incubated in an atmosphere of reduced oxygen tension attained by the following methods: candle jar, gas generating kits with and without active catalyst. The candle jar method, which is easy, cheap and simple, is recommended for the isolation of **C. jejuni** in this environment.

Imported campylobacter, shigella and salmonella infections in Finland

T. Pitkanen,* T. U. Kosunen,† M. Jahkola,§ A. Ponka* and T. Pettersson*

*Department of Medicine and Tropical Diseases, Aurora Hospital; †Department of Bacteriology and Immunology, University of Helsinki, and §Public Health Institute, Helsinki, Finland

Campylobacter jejuni was isolated from the faeces of 19 (5.8%) out of 329 travellers with diarrhoea, treated as outpatients at the Tropical Outpatients Department of Aurora Hospital. During an 18-month period these travellers, together with 446 other diarrhoeal patients, showed a 7.1% incidence of campylobacter enteritis. Eighty-five per cent (47 of 55) of these cases were imported, whereas the frequency in all of Finland during a three-year period was 52% (369 of 712).

The traveller's risk of contracting campylobacter enteritis varied from country to country, being highest in Morocco and Tunisia (29 and 16.4 per 10,000 travellers). Risk averaged 1.5 per 10,000, based on 43 countries and 2,443,000 travellers, with Portugal (3.9), Romania (2.1) and Bulgaria (1.7) also rising above the mean. Risk was from 1.3 to 0.4 in Spain, Poland, the USSR, Greece and Italy.

The traveller's risk of contracting shigella infection varied from country to country following the pattern of campylobacter enteritis, but a remarkably large proportion of shigella infections, 63% (244 of 387), was imported from 10 observed tourist countries compared to that of campylobacter enteritis, 26% (95 of 369). Multiresistant strains of shigella were not imported from Morocco or Tunisia. Multiresistant strains of shigella and campylobacter were recognised from the Far East.

In the salmonella group the pattern of 10 countries remained to an extent, but was scattered by epidemics. Altogether **Salmonella typhimurium** proves to be mainly a domestic problem, with 25% imported infections, but in other infections travel outside Scandinavia was the cause of 52% in campylobacter, 64% in salmonella "alia" (excluding **S. typhimurium**, and including five imported **S. typhi** infections out of a total of nine) and 93% in shigella cases in Finland over three years. The figures presented give a rational basis for allocating surveillance measures in campylobacter, shigella and salmonella infections in Finland.

Faecal carriage of Campylobacter jejuni among workers at chicken processing plants, Santiago, Chile

A. Soto, **G. Figueroa**, M. Troncoso and S. Urcelay

Instituto de Nutricion y Technologia de los Alimentos, Universidad de Chile, Casilla 15138, Santiago 11, Chile

Studies of the prevalence of faecal carriage of **Campylobacter jejuni** in poultry in both industrialised and less-developed countries have revealed high rates. This implies that workers in poultry processing plants who manipulate the birds may be at increased risk of acquiring **C. jejuni** infection. In an attempt to assess this, 115 workers in three chicken processing plants in Santiago were studied with a health status questionnaire and a rectal swab culture.

The workers studied came from four sections of the processing line with varying degrees of direct manipulation of chickens. The highest prevalence of **C. jejuni** was 7% (eight of 115 workers). The overall prevalence was in eviscerators (six of 51, 12%), followed by those who bled (one of 22, 5%), dressed carcasses (one of 32, 3%) or refrigerated the processed meat (none of 10, 0%). The rate in eviscerators (six of 51) was significantly higher than in the other workers (three of 64, 3%) (P = 0.06). Diarrhoea was reported significantly more often in workers infected with **C. jejuni** (six of eight, 75%) than in uninfected individuals (33 of 107, 31%) (P = 0.017). In contrast, no correlation was found between diarrhoea and **C. coli** infection. **C. jejuni** infection represents an occupational hazard for workers in processing plants who manipulate poultry directly.

Campylobacters in children in Vietnam

F. Megraud and Pham Cue Kanh

Paediatric Hospital No. 2, Ho Chi Minh City, Vietnam

During a one-month period in April 1983 (hot, dry season) we looked for campylobacters in the faeces of 375 children (0–15 years old) hospitalised with enteric infections in Ho Chi Minh City. A control group of 92 children without intestinal disorders, age matched, was chosen from children in different day-care centres and schools in the city. The age distribution of the children was as follows: 0–1 year, 41%; 1–3 years, 34%; 3–5 years, 11.5%; 5–10 years, 8%; 10–15 years, 5.5%.

The selective medium used was Butzler's medium (Virion). The plates were incubated at 42 °C for 24–48 h in microaerobic conditions, which were the culture conditions used in similar studies in France (see p. 150).

In the patient group, seven campylobacters were found (1.9%) in addition to 31 rotaviruses, 27 salmonellae, 14 shigellae and two **Vibrio cholerae** O1. Three campylobacters and two salmonellae were found in the control group. Nine of the 10 campylobacter strains were characterised as

Campylobacter coli and had different sensitivities to metranidazole and TTC by comparison with the French swine strains.

This low incidence of campylobacter infection may be related to season. During the monsoon period the incidence is increased to 5%. An alternative explanation may be the lack of milk and meat consumption in the population under study. Further research needs to be carried out to confirm this preliminary result.

4. Animal and environmental sources

Field studies on campylobacter infections in domestic animals

L. Roberts, M. C. Allan, E. J. Walker and D. K. Sommerville

Veterinary Investigation Laboratory, Mill of Craibstone, Bucksburn, Aberdeen AB2 9TS, UK

For over three years, material submitted to the Veterinary Investigation Laboratory from the Grampian Region of Scotland has been examined for the presence of **Campylobacter** spp. Campylobacters have been recovered from all species of bird and animal examined to date. **C. jejuni** is very common in the sheep population, with **C. fetus** subsp. **fetus** less commonly recovered. In cattle, thermophilic campylobacters, **C. fetus** subsp. **fetus** and **C. hyointestinalis** are all commonly isolated.

Serotyping of sheep and cattle isolates belonging to the thermophilic groups, based on the heat-stable antigens and using the PHA technique of Penner and Hennessey, has shown that the following serotypes are commonest.

(1) In sheep, 61% of typable isolates belong to one of the five groups 4,13,16,34,43,50; 1,44; 23,36; 2; 1.

(2) In cattle, 58% of typable isolates belong to one of the four groups 4,13,16,34,43,50; 2; 24; 23.

The 4,13,16,34,43,50 strain is common in both the bovine and the ovine populations and included here are strains which may lack one or two of these antigenic determinants.

In a longitudinal study in a beef suckler herd in which cows and calves have been sampled on a regular basis for over two years, all the main types of campylobacter found in the cattle populations are present: thermophilic campylobacters (predominantly **C. jejuni** biotype 1), **C. fetus** subsp. **fetus** and **C. hyointestinalis**. During the period of study all three organisms have been maintained within the group and on occasions campylobacters are recoverable from almost all the animals in the group.

To study the epidemiology of campylobacter infections in dairy herds, 12 herds are being sampled monthly for a 12 month period. All 12 herds have been infected with campylobacters at every sampling. **C. jejuni** biotype 1 has been the commonest isolate, but **C. jejuni** biotype 2, **C. coli**, **C. laridis**, **C. fetus** subsp. **fetus** and **C. hyointestinalis** have been recovered. Of the thermophilic campylobacter isolates typed to date, 85% of the typable isolates belonged to one of the following six types: 23,26; 4,13,16,34,43,50; 1,44; 11; 8,17; 2.

Isolation of Campylobacter jejuni from animals in Zaire

L. R. Van Damme* and S. Lauwers†

*Laboratoire Veterinaire, BP 8842, Kinshasa X, Zaire, and †Infectious Disease Unit, Free University of Brussels, Brussels, Belgium

De Mol and Bosmans confirmed the pathogenicity of **Campylobacter jejuni** in children with diarrhoea in Kigali (Rwanda, Central Africa), but little is known about animal carriage of **C. jejuni** in Central Africa.

We investigated the carriage rate of **C. jejuni** in 224 animals in Zaire (region of Kinshasa) from December 1981 to April 1983. Samples (faeces and pieces of intestine) were inoculated on Butzler's medium and incubated at a temperature of 42 °C, for 48–72 h, in an anaerobic jar without a catalyst and with a gas generating kit.

We isolated **C. jejuni** from 65 animals (29% of the total number examined). The highest isolation rates were found in pigs, with 42 (44%) positive out of 95 examined, and in chickens, with 14 (38%) positive out of 36 examined. We did not isolate **C. jejuni** from 64 cattle, three dogs and one monkey. The other animals studied were five sheep (two positive), 11 ducks (three positive) and nine birds from zoological gardens (four positive).

In pigs the youngest animals (weanling pigs of less than 2 months old) were more frequently positive than the older ones: 13 positive out of 19 examined for the weanlings and 25 positive out of 72 examined for the older group.

Fifteen **C. jejuni** isolates were serotyped: 10 pig strains and five chicken strains. Five strains were untypable; the remaining 10 strains belonged to nine different serotypes, two of which are common in Europe (LAU 1 and LAU 6).

Isolation, characterisation and serotyping of Campylobacter jejuni and Campylobacter coli from slaughter cattle

M. M. Garcia,* H. Lior,† R. B. Stewart,* G. M. Ruckerbauer* and A. Skljarevski§

*Agriculture Canada, Animal Diseases Research Institute, PO Box 11300, Station H, Nepean, Ontario K2H 8P9; †National Enteric Reference Center, Bureau of Microbiology, Laboratory Center for Disease Control, Ottawa, Ontario K1A 0L2; and §Crabtree Meat Packers, PO Box 7028, Vanier, Ontario K1L 8E2, Canada

Some 525 specimens were obtained from 100 slaughter beef cattle and examined for the presence of **Campylobacter jejuni** and **C. coli** by direct plating and enrichment techniques. Isolates were identified by cultural, biochemical, immunofluorescence and antibiotic susceptibility tests and further characterised with the aid of recent biotyping and serotyping schemes. Fifty animals were positive for **C. jejuni** and one was positive for **C. coli**. The distribution pattern of positive animals, in decreasing order, was steers (57%), bulls (40%), heifers (40%) and cows (22%). Significantly higher isolation rates were obtained from the gallbladders (34%), large intestines (36%) and small intestines (32%) than from liver (12%) or lymph nodes (1.4%). Isolations from the enrichment techniques were 42% more than from direct plating; 24 h enrichment resulted in 24% more isolations then 48 h enrichment.

Eighty-one of 103 cultures were typable serologically and represented 14 serotypes. Serotype 7 was most commonly encountered (35%), followed by serotypes 5 (12%) and 1 (8%). Each of the remaining 11 serotypes accounted for 1-6% of the typable cultures. These results provide further evidence that serotypes commonly isolated from human sources are also encountered in cattle.

Campylobacter jejuni epidemiology in broiler production: the reality of campylobacter-free flocks

S. Shanker,* A. Lee† and T. C. Sorrell§

*Bacteriology Department, Institute of Clinical Pathology and Medical Research, Westmead Centre, Westmead, New South Wales 2145, Australia; †School of Microbiology, University of New South Wales, PO Box 1, Kensington, Australia; and §Infectious Diseases Unit, Westmead Centre, and Department of Medicine, University of Sydney, New South Wales, Australia

Despite many reports of contamination of processed broilers by **Campylobacter jejuni**, research on the source of this bacterium has been limited. In this epidemiological study, broiler flocks in two districts (A and B) were monitored for **C. jejuni**.

Cloacal swabs were obtained from 27 flocks at 15 grow-out farms and three flocks at one breeder farm. In district A, the incidence of **C. jejuni** in grow-out farms was low (one of 10 farms). Broilers at the "positive" farm were 6 weeks old. The organism was isolated from cloacal swabs and water but not feed or litter. Flocks from the same parent farm placed in this "positive" farm after it was cleaned remained free of **C. jejuni**.

Important findings relevant to **C. jejuni** transmission were obtained in the breeder farm which supplied eggs to the common hatchery for the grow-out farms. At the breeder farm two flocks aged 34 and 39 weeks were "positive". A third flock at this farm became "positive" within 5 weeks of introduction, indicating horizontal transmission. However, none of the eight flocks of broilers, which were stocked from the contaminated breeder farm via the hatchery, showed any "positive" birds, suggesting that vertical transmission via eggs is unlikely. In district B, broiler flocks in four of five farms were "positive". The age of these birds ranged from 2 to 6 weeks. Differences in environmental conditions and husbandry practices in these two districts are being investigated, together with the ability of **C. jejuni** to survive in farm water, litter and feed under various conditions.

Campylobacter jejuni in poultry processing and pig slaughtering

J. Oosterom* and G. J. A. de Wilde†

*National Institute of Public Health, Laboratory for Zoonoses and Food Microbiology, PO Box 1, 3720 BA Bilthoven, and †Meat Inspection Service, Anjelierstraat 2, 7641 CG Wierden, The Netherlands

Investigations were carried out to determine prevalence and survival of **Campylobacter jejuni** in poultry processing plants and in pig slaughterhouses.

Broiler chickens that are transported to processing plants may carry many campylobacters in the intestinal tract (mean number 10^4 c.f.u./g, maximum 10^7 c.f.u./g). Examination of pieces of pericloacal skin from chickens in different stages of processing showed that this intestinal colonisation with **C. jejuni** may be responsible for all contamination found along the processing line. **C. jejuni** was not eliminated during scalding of the birds (maximum D-value at 58 °C is 0.39 min, and at 52 °C is more than 10 min), and numbers returned to initial levels after defeathering and evisceration. Large numbers of **C. jejuni** were also found in processing water (maximum 10^3 c.f.u./ml) and in the air in processing halls (maximum 10^4 c.f.u./m^3). Some 50–75% of end-products were contaminated. In many instances cooling of poultry end-products did not reduce the contamination.

Pigs are also frequent carriers of campylobacters but, in general, pork seems to have a very low contamination rate. It was found that almost total elimination of campylobacter on pig carcasses occurs when they are cooled in the slaughterhouse. Experiments in the laboratory showed that this elimination is not caused by low temperatures, but is due to the drying effect of the forced ventilation used in abattoir cooling rooms. Campylobacters appeared to be very sensitive to drying.

Campylobacter jejuni in broilers, hens and eggs in a developing country

G. Figueroa, H. Hidalgo, M. Troncoso, S. Rosende and V. Soto

Instituto de Nutricion y Tecnologia de los Alimentos (INTA) and Escuela de Ciencias Veterinarias, Universidad de Chile, Casilla 15138, Santiago 11, Chile

Some animal species serve as reservoirs for **Campylobacter jejuni**, an enteropathogen for man. To evaluate the role of poultry as a potential source for human infection, the frequency of isolation and antimicrobial sensitivity of **C. jejuni** were studied. **C. jejuni** was detected in 96% of cloacal samples from 26 live broilers, 84% of 25 processed birds ready for sale, 55% of 200 caged laying hens and 25% of 200 freshly laid eggs. Cultures from eggs were performed from swabbing on their surfaces and from homogenates of shells and membranes. Six samples of drinking water from one laying hen farm were also studied: two of them grew **C. jejuni**. In addition, when salmonellae were surveyed simultaneously in the laying hens, eggs and drinking water only **Salmonella typhimurium** var. Copenhagen was cultured from 10% of the hens and eggs and from one of the water samples. Reistance to tetracycline and erythromycin in **C. jejuni** isolates from hens was 73% and 18% respectively; for eggs these proportions were 60% and 40%; for water 50% and 0%; for live broilers 35% and 20%. By contrast, all strains isolated from processed broilers were susceptible to both antibiotics. **C. jejuni** recovery rates were high in all sources investigated, and in only one case was it associated with salmonellae. In our environment, appropriate handling and cooking of chickens and eggs appear as important steps in reducing the risk of human infection.

Campylobacter infection: an occupational disease risk in chicken handlers

O. Grados,* **N. Bravo,*** J. P. Butzler† and G. Ventura*

*National Enteropathogens Reference Laboratory, National Institute of Health, Lima, Peru, and †Laboratoire de Microbiologie, Hopital Universitaire St Pierre, Bruxelles, Belgium

Eighty chicken handlers in a market in Lima (Linca) were studied bacteriologically for **Campylobacter jejuni**. The same number of non-chicken handlers, from the same market, were sampled as a control group.

Samples from 160 chickens were obtained. Chickens arrive at the market alive and are killed and eviscerated before sale. Samples were obtained by swabbing the cloaca of live chickens and the bodies of chickens ready for sale.

Results showed 15 persons (19%) positive for **C. jejuni** among handlers and none positive among the control group (P = 0.000029). Some 136 (85%) out of 160 chickens were positive for **C. jejuni**. It is considered that chicken handlers have a higher risk of infection and are carriers of **C. jejuni**. Consequently the chicken handlers are potential transmitters of this infection to a susceptible population.

Campylobacter jejuni in game and poultry (other than chicken)

E. de Boer,* G. J. A. de Wilde† and B. J. Hartog§

*Food Inspection Service, PO Box 9012, 7200 GN Zutphen; †Meat Inspection Service, Anjelierstraat 2, 7641 CG Wierden; and §Food Inspection Service, PO Box 777, 7500 AT Enschede, The Netherlands

The intestinal contents of a number of animals, shot during hunting or obtained from a rearing farm, were surveyed for the presence of **Campylobacter jejuni**. Samples from a turkey and a domestic duck slaughterhouse, and carcasses of several animals from retail sources were also included in the study. **C. jejuni** was isolated from two of 25 hares, three of 21 wild boars, six of 49 pheasants, 19 of 88 wild ducks, two of 16 wild geese and nine of 25 wood-pigeons, but from none of eight partridges. From one of the **C. jejuni** positive hares, **C. jejuni** was isolated in high numbers from both the intestinal contents and the liver; swabs from the peritoneal cavity were also **C. jejuni** positive. The hare was very lean and ill-looking. Possibly these symptoms were caused by the campylobacter infection. The **C. jejuni**-positive wild boars were shot in an area where these animals were fed from offal from a poultry slaughterhouse. Fourteen of 20 pheasants and all of 10 guinea fowls from a rearing farm were positive for **C. jejuni**, as were 22 of 26 samples of neck skin of turkeys from three turkey slaughterhouses. Samples were taken on five different days in a domestic duck slaughterhouse: on four days **C. jejuni** was isolated from duck carcasses, eviscerators and spinchiller water, but on one day swabs from 12 duck carcasses were **C. jejuni**-negative, which indicates that **C. jejuni**-negative flocks occur.

Samples of frozen carcasses from retail sources were surveyed for the presence of **C. jejuni**: one of 25 pheasants, one of 17 guinea fowls and three of 19 turkeys were **C. jejuni**-positive, but **C. jejuni** could not be isolated from 19 wild and 22 domestic rabbits, 24 wood-pigeons, 16 wild ducks and seven hares. The low contamination levels of these products was probably caused by the sensitivity of **C. jejuni** to freezing.

Possible sources of contamination of game and poultry with **C. jejuni** are as follows: (a) ingestion of contaminated food; (b) contamination of the living animals through the environment by way of contaminated surface water, birds, rodents, insects, etc.; (c) cross-contamination during the slaughterhouse process; (d) insufficiently hygienic handling of the shot animals after hunting (e.g. contamination of carcasses with intestinal contents, soil or water; inadequate protection of shot animals against vermin, predators and hounds; contamination during transport and cross-contamination in the retail trade).

Wild birds as Campylobacter vectors in the agricultural environment

D. R. Fenlon

Bacteriology Division, School of Agriculture, University of Aberdeen, Aberdeen, UK

A study of the carriage of campylobacters by those bird species which congregate on pastures used by livestock has shown the proportion of birds harbouring the organism to be high (gulls 10–67%; pigeons 25–40%; geese 10–60%; rooks 45–83%), with numbers of the organisms often in excess of 10^6 per gram of faeces. In view of the evidence for a low infective dose, these levels of carriage and excretion may constitute a significant reservoir of infection.

The parallels with the transmission of salmonellas are obvious; birds have been implicated in a number of outbreaks of salmonellosis in cattle and sheep in Scotland and both groups of organisms have been responsible for large scale outbreaks of milk-borne disease in recent years.

The biotypes of campylobacters carried by birds do not appear to be related to their feeding habits. A variety of biotypes is found in gulls, whereas in rooks, pigeons and geese, the principal human pathogen,

Campylobacter jejuni biotype 1, predominates, and so these latter vectors may present the greater risk.

In some bird species which consume very large quantities of low energy foodstuffs, for example geese, grazing on grass, the faeces may show few or no coliform bacteria, yet campylobacters can be isolated. There are circumstances, therefore, when the coliform test may not be a reliable indicator of the potential presence of faecal pathogens such as **C. jejuni.**

The role of Larus gulls in the epidemiology of campylobacters in Scotland

C. R. Fricker

Scottish Salmonella Reference Laboratory, Department of Bacteriology, Stobhill General Hospital, Springburn, Glasgow G21 3UW, UK

The occurrence of campylobacters in the intestinal tract of wild birds is well known, and it has been suggested that avian contamination of water supplies could lead to human infection. The population of seagulls (**Larus** spp.) has been increasing steadily this century at an annual rate of 13% and now stands at over one million birds.

A comparison of procedures for the isolation of campylobacters from seagull faecal material [1] showed that enrichment was a vital part of technique and that a system of enrichment in Preston broth [2] followed by plating on Preston agar [2] led to the highest number of isolations.

A national survey of some 3126 gulls showed that 2492 (80.0%) were carrying campylobacters and 218 (7.0%) salmonellae. Table 1 shows the distribution of campylobacter "biotypes" obtained from the gulls.

Table 1 The distribution of campylobacter "biotypes" isolated from 3126 seagulls captured in Scotland

	Herring gull	Lesser black-backed gull
C. jejuni type 1	461 (21.3%)	198 (20.6%)
C. jejuni type 2	213 (9.8%)	94 (9.8%)
C. coli	250 (11.6%)	117 (12.1%)
C. laridis (NARTC)	741 (34.3%)	323 (33.5%)
NARTC H_2S negative	68 (3.1%)	27 (2.8%)
No campylobacters isolated	430 (19.9%)	204 (21.2%)
Total	2163	963

Table 2 The number of salmonella and campylobacter isolates from 3126 gulls captured in various regions of Scotland

	Total examined	Salmonella positive	Campylobacter positive
West Scotland (Glasgow area)	1455	149 (10.2%)	1164 (80.0%)
West Scotland (rural)	275	25 (9.1%)	218 (79.3%)
North Scotland (rural)	411	8 (1.9%)	322 (78.3%)
East Scotland (urban)	362	23 (6.4%)	294 (81.2%)
East Scotland (rural)	623	13 (2.1%)	494 (79.3%)
Total	3126	218 (7.0%)	2495 (79.7%)

Table 2 shows the number of salmonella and campylobacter isolates from different geographical locations in Scotland. Whilst the occurrence of salmonella in the gulls was markedly affected by the site of capture, no such geographical variation was seen with the isolation of campylobacters.

REFERENCES

1. C. R. Fricker, R. W. A. Girdwood and D. Munro. A comparison of procedures for the isolation of campylobacters from seagull faeces. Journal of Hygiene, Cambridge, 1983, in press.
2. F. J. Bolton and L. Robertson. A selective medium for isolating **Campylobacter jejuni/coli**. Journal of Clinical Pathology, 1982, **35**, 462-467.

Seasonal study of a freshwater lake for Campylobacter jejuni

G. A. Hill and D. J. Grimes

Department of Biology and River Studies Center, University of Wisconsin-La Crosse, La Crosse, Wisconsin 54601, USA

In the summer and fall of 1981, water and sediment samples from Lake Onalaska, a Mississippi River navigation pool, were quantitatively examined for **Campylobacter jejuni** and for standard bacterial indicators of fecal pollution. Fifty cecal samples, representing seven species of transient waterfowl captured during fall migration, were also assayed for **C. jejuni.** Fecal coliform and fecal streptococcus counts from the water and sediment samples agreed with previously established values for the pool and accurately reflected the influx of ducks and geese during fall migration. **C. jejuni** was not isolated from water, sediment or cecal samples. This conflicts with previous reports which implied a cosmopolitan distribution of **C. jejuni** among waterfowl. Reasons for the absence of **C. jejuni** from the pool and from waterfowl impacting that pool are discussed, with special reference to survival of the organism, method of recovery, correlation with water quality parameters, and sporadic distribution of other pathogens among migratory waterfowl.

Campylobacters isolated from the environment and from patients in Hull and East Yorkshire

S. L. Mawer

Public Health Laboratory, Hull Royal Infirmary, Anlaby Road, Hull HU3 2JZ, UK

Many of the patients with campylobacter enteritis in Hull were noted to live close to the numerous land drains and water courses present within the city boundary. A regular weekly sampling programme of the ponds, lakes and land drains was therefore carried out with the help of the Kingston-upon-Hull Environmental Health Department to determine whether or not campylobacters were present in these waters and to see if there was any correlation between the types found in the water and those in patients.

Specimens of water from ponds, lakes and land-drains within Hull and from the River Hull were examined by a membrane isolation technique on to Preston medium. The isolates from patients and from water were identified by methods described by Skirrow and were serotyped by Manchester Public Health Laboratory.

Most of the human strains (86%) were identified as **Campylobacter jejuni** (hippurate positive, TTC sensitive, compared with a **C. jejuni** control) whereas most of the environmental strains (73%) were hippurate negative but TTC sensitive compared with a **C. jejuni** control. There were many antigens, as demonstrated by the Penner system, shared between the human and environmental strains.

Human volunteer experiments were then performed to determine the pathogenicity of the strains that were likely to be taken into the water treatment plant serving East Hull by drinking that water.

EXPERIMENT 1   200 ml of water from the River Hull near a trout farm, where the water is clean and unpolluted, contained between 10 and 100 non-typable campylobacters which were nalidixic acid sensitive, hippurate negative, TTC sensitive compared with a **C. jejuni** control. No symptoms were experienced.

EXPERIMENT 2   Same source. No campylobacters isolated from 100 ml. No symptoms.

EXPERIMENT 3   400 ml of water from River Hull at Bell Mills, Driffield. The water contained MPN > 11,000 per 10 ml campylobacters which were nalidixic sensitive, hippurate negative and TTC sensitive compared with a **C. jejuni** control. Of 13 isolates tested, one belonged to type 4, two to type 28(weak), one to type 28(weak),39, one to type 28(weak),39(weak), one to 39(weak) and seven were non-typable. No symptoms were experienced.

Faecal specimens were plated on and enriched in Preston media. Sera were examined for the presence of campylobacter antibodies by Manchester Public Health Laboratory. No campylobacters were isolated and no antibodies were detected to the strains ingested in Experiment 3.

CONCLUSIONS (1) The campylobacters isolated from the environment are biochemically different from human strains. (2) Ingestion from natural water containing > 11,000 environmental campylobacters did not produce symptoms or a detectable antibody response. (3) Treated water from this river is unlikely to have been the source of infection in the Hull cases. (4) The association of cases with ponds and land-drains in the city probably occurred by chance.

A prospective epidemiological study of campylobacters from a river and the adjoining meadow

M. S. Khan

Pathology Laboratory, Lakin Road, Warwick CV34 5BJ, UK

A three-year survey was set up from January 1980 to December 1982 to study the prevalence and distribution of thermophilic campylobacters from the environment around a river bank and its adjoining meadow. This meadow is often flooded and wild ducks and various waterfowl breed nearby. Large flocks of seagulls also rest and feed there. It is also a popular place for the residents to exercise their dogs. The purpose of the study was to establish whether there was a correlation between the prevalence and time of appearance of certain serotypes of thermophilic campylobacters and the outbreak of campylobacter enteritis in a number of dogs and people living in the adjoining area.

Every fortnight, 25 samples were taken for culture: three of river bank mud, two of river water, 10 of dog excreta and 10 of fowl droppings from the nesting area and river bank.

In the first year of the study (1980), there was an outbreak of campylobacter enteritis affecting dogs and humans in the second week of July after a sudden rise in the isolation rate of the same serotype (Manchester 3 = Lior 4 = Penner 2) from the environment.

In the second year (1981), there was a correspondingly increased isolation rate during the summer months of one NARTC serotype which was consequently proved to be **Campylobacter laridis** [1]. This increase was first observed in the seagull droppings but later on it spread equally into all environmental samples. Yet no cases of enteritis in either humans or dogs came to light during 1981.

In the third year (1982), there was no increase in any one particular serotype of thermophilic campylobacter until early September, when one serotype (Manchester 2 = Lior 1 = Penner 4) became prevalent. A month earlier, the same serotype had been isolated from two newly acquired puppies and later on from one adult dog from the neighbourhood. All the three dogs had diarrhoea.

The results of the study suggest that the immediate environment with its wildfowl may be acting as a reservoir of human infection. The prevalence and time of appearance of certain serotypes seem to be associated with human and dog infections, whereas in the case of **C. laridis** no such associated outbreak was observed.

REFERENCE

1. J. Benjamin, S. Leaper, R. J. Owen and M. B. Skirrow: Description of **Campylobacter laridis**, a new species comprising the nalidixic acid resistant thermophilic campylobacter (NARTC) group. Current Microbiology, 1983, **8**, 231-238.

Isolation of thermophilic campylobacters from houseflies

O. Rosef* and G. Kapperud*†

*Institute of Food Hygiene, The Norwegian College of Veterinary Medicine, and †Norwegian Defence Microbiological Laboratory, Oslo, Norway

Adult houseflies (**Musca domestica**) are important agents in the dissemination of numerous infectious diseases. In this study, 161 strains of thermophilic campylobacters were isolated from 608 houseflies in Norway. A majority of the isolates (90.1%) belonged to **Campylobacter coli**, followed by **C. jejuni** (6.2%) and nalidixic acid-resistant thermophilic campylobacters (NARTC) (3.7%). Isolates were obtained from 50.7% of flies captured on a chicken farm and 43.2% of flies from a piggery.

Thirty-eight strains were serotyped on the basis of heat-stable antigens (Lauwers' serotype scheme). The typable strains fell into 14 different serotypes, four of which have previously been isolated from human patients in Norway. Some 66.7% of the campylobacters isolated from flies inhabiting a piggery belonged to common porcine serotypes, whereas 47.1% of the campylobacters isolated from flies from a chicken farm belonged to serotypes previously isolated from poultry. Three flies harboured biochemically distinct strains (**C. jejuni** and NARTC). It is probable that flies transmit campylobacters from domestic animals to man, or vice versa, and between different species of animal. It is also conceivable that flies could introduce the pathogen into herds or flocks of domestic animals previously free from campylobacters.

The isolation of Campylobacter jejuni from flies

E. P. Wright

Public Health Laboratory, Luton and Dunstable Hospital, Lewsey Road, Luton LU4 0DZ, UK [Present address: Department of Microbiology, Royal East Sussex Hospital, Cambridge Road, Hastings, East Sussex TN34 1ER, UK]

Although it is well known that enteropathogenic bacteria are carried by flies, there are few reports of the isolation of **Campylobacter jejuni** from flies. Rosef and Kapperud [1] in Norway reported the isolation of **C. jejuni** from 28.4% of houseflies. The aim of the present study was to determine the incidence of **C. jejuni** in flies collected in Britain.

Between May and September 1982 a total of 259 flies were caught in domestic houses and gardens. At first, pooled collections of between two and 10 flies were cultured as one sample; later individual flies were examined. The samples were cultured by direct and enrichment methods using Preston selective medium incubated under appropriate conditions.

Of 18 pooled samples examined (total of 49 flies) **C. jejuni** was isolated from one sample containing nine flies. A total of 210 flies were examined individually; five (2.4%) yielded **C. jejuni**. Altogether, seven strains of **C. jejuni** were isolated; one fly yielded two distinct strains. The distribution of biotypes was as follows: **C. jejuni** biotype 1, two; **C. jejuni** biotype 2, three; and **C. coli**, two.

The difference in isolation rates between this study and that of Rosef and Kapperud is that in the present study flies were collected in houses and gardens away from farms and abattoirs, whereas in the Norwegian study the culture-positive flies were collected from a chicken farm and piggery and therefore could have had more access to infected animal faeces. In addition, the survival time of **C. jejuni** either as a surface contaminant or in the alimentary tract of the fly has yet to be determined, so that the flies in the present study may have been carrying **C. jejuni** which were no longer viable.

REFERENCE

1. O. Rosef and G. Kapperud. Houseflies (**Musca domestica**) as possible vectors of **Campylobacter fetus** subsp. **jejuni**. Applied and Environmental Microbiology 1983, **45**, 381-383.

Do campylobacters contaminate food preparation areas?

D. N. Hutchinson, H. C. Dawkins and F. J. Bolton

Public Health Laboratory, Royal Infirmary, Meadow Street, Preston PR1 6PS, UK

Four food kitchens preparing chickens for consumption by large groups of people were studied to assess the environmental contamination by **Campylobacter** spp.:

(1) Hospital kitchen, preparing batches of 20-40 chickens.
(2) University kitchen, preparing batches of 20-100 fresh or frozen chickens.
(3) Cook-freeze unit, in which batches of 100 frozen chickens are processed. After cooking birds are blast-frozen, portioned and plated, and stored frozen until distribution.

(4) Commercial roast-chicken unit, i.e. a large kitchen processing approximately 2000 fresh and frozen chickens daily. After steam-roasting the birds are blast-frozen, portioned and packed for the catering trade.

Each kitchen was visited on four occasions. Samples were taken of chicken carcasses and giblets, and the working surfaces, sinks and hands of kitchen personnel were swabbed before and during processing. After cleaning of surfaces, further swabs were collected.

Campylobacters were not isolated from the environment of any kitchen before processing.

On 10 visits campylobacter organisms were isolated from carcass swabs, and on six of these visits campylobacters were isolated from the surrounding work surfaces during processing. Surfaces were found to be contaminated on one occasion when organisms were not detected on carcasses or giblets.

A higher proportion of isolations was made by swabbing the insides of the carcasses as opposed to the outer surfaces. Thawed juices and giblets were a frequent source of campylobacters. **Campylobacter** spp. were isolated from the operator's hands on two of 12 occasions after preparation but not after washing.

COMMENT Contamination of the hands and work surfaces occurs frequently whilst preparing raw chickens. Cleaning with detergents and hot water is adequate for removal of organisms from the working environment.

B. SURVIVAL EXPERIMENTS

Inactivation of pathogens in sewage by irradiation with special reference to Campylobacter jejuni

M. M. Garcia,* B. W. Brooks,* R. B. Stewart* and T. Ouwerkerk†

*Animal Diseases Research Institute, 801 Fallowfield Road, PO Box 11300, Station H, Nepean, Ontario K2H 8P9, and †Atomic Energy of Canada Ltd, Commercial Products, PO Box 6300, Ottawa, Ontario K2A 3W3, Canada

Sewage samples from animal wastes and effluents from an animal disease laboratory were spiked with known numbers of pathogenic organisms and subjected to various doses of gamma irradiation from a ^{60}Co source. Surviving test organisms were quantitatively determined by selective and enrichment techniques. The dose response of **Campylobacter jejuni** appeared to be linear throughout inactivation. The D_{10} value, that is the irradiation dose necessary to reduce the population by one $\log_{10}$, was approximately 0.02 Mrad for **C. jejuni** in animal sewage. No significant difference was observed whether the sewage was of bovine or poultry origin. However, the D_{10} value in the laboratory effluent was approximately 10 times lower. The rating of the test organisms in decreasing order of radio-sensitivity was as follows: **Brucella abortus, Campylobacter jejuni, Mycobacterium fortuitum, Candida albicans, Clostridium difficile** and **Streptococcus faecalis.**

Survival of thermophilic campylobacters in water

B. Gondrosen

Institute of Food Hygiene, The Norwegian College of Veterinary Medicine, Olso, Norway

The survival of **Campylobacter jejuni** (one strain of serotype LAU 1,27), **C. coli** (one strain of serotype LAU 8,11) and **C. laridis** (NARTC) (one strain of serotype LAU 14) in water was studied. Standard inocula were added to (i) chlorinated tap water, (ii) unchlorinated tap water, (iii) polluted river water, (iv) sterile filtered river water, or (v) physiological saline, and kept at 4, 12 or 20 °C. Samples were withdrawn daily to determine viable counts. Ten millilitres of water were doubly filtered through (a) a Millipore 450 nm HC filter, followed by (b) a Millipore 200 nm filter. Both filters were placed on two selective agar plates: colimycin-amphotericin-keflin (CAK) agar and Skirrow's agar. Incubation was at 42 °C for 24 and 48 h in a microaerophilic atmosphere. The results were as follows:

(1) All organisms survived better at 4 °C than at 12 or 20 °C in all media tested. Briefest survival was obtained at 20 °C; no viable bacteria could be detected after 2 days at this temperature in any of the media.

(2) Maximum viability was 21 days for **C. jejuni** in physiological saline kept at 4 °C. **C. coli** and **C. laridis** survived for only 5 days in this medium (12 °C).

(3) All strains remained viable for 15 days in unchlorinated tap water at 4 °C (10 days at 12 °C). Chlorination (0.1 mg Cl per litre) drastically reduced the survival of all three strains examined; **C. coli** and NARTC died within 1 day in chlorinated tap water, whereas **C. jejuni** remained viable for 4 days at 4 °C (3 days at 12 °C).

(4) All strains survived for 10-15 days in polluted river water at 4 °C (6-12 days at 12 °C). Removal of interspecific competition by sterile filtration did not significantly enhance survival.

Some factors affecting the spread of Campylobacter jejuni by foods

R. W. A. Park and S. C. Waterman*

Microbiology Department, Reading University, London Road, Reading RG1 5AQ, UK [*Present address: G. D. Searle & Co. Ltd, PO Box 53, Lane End Road, High Wycombe, Buckinghamshire HP12 4HL, UK]

The apparent inability of **Campylobacter jejuni** to grow below 30 °C and the reported small infective dose mean that concern about the organism in food centres on the opportunities for and extent of contamination of food and on the ability of the organism to survive once in the food. Cattle faeces and chicken are acknowledged sources of the organism. Experiments have been undertaken in which **C. jejuni** has been added to foods and other materials and its survival assessed by making counts after various periods. **C. jejuni** died so rapidly during the manufacture of soft cheese that its spread by cheese made from contaminated milk is highly improbable. The possiblity of cross-contamination occurring via work surfaces (simulated by glass slides) and wiping cloths (simulated by pieces of cloth) was demonstrated by adding drops of suspension of **C. jejuni** to these items at 25 °C. The organisms survived sufficiently well for spread by these agents to be important (decimal reduction time of between 0.5 h and 1 day). More than 10% of the organisms inoculated into raw minced beef survived for 3 days at 4 °C. Survival on various cooked meats at 4 °C was good, with a decimal reduction time of several days.

The survival of Campylobacter jejuni in milk

D. W. Redwood, K. P. W. Gill and **K. P. Lander**

Ministry of Agriculture, Fisheries and Food, Central Veterinary Laboratory, New Haw, Weybridge, Surrey KT15 3NB, UK

Bovine and human isolates of **Campylobacter jejuni** remained viable in sterile milk for periods of 8–146 days at 4 °C and 3–49 days at ambient temperature.

A single strain retained a viable count of 10^7 for 15 days in ultra-high-temperature (UHT) treated milk at ambient temperature and at pH 6.0. The strain was killed in 30 min by acidified water at pH 5.0, whereas acidified broth allowed it to survive for 24 h.

It was shown that milk has fairly strong buffering power and that volumes of more than 150 ml of milk will neutralise the gastric acid present in normal human stomach.

Effect of various gas atmospheres on the growth or survival of Campylobacter jejuni on meat

M.-L. Hanninen,* H. Korkeala* and P. Pakkala†

*College of Veterinary Medicine, Department of Food Hygiene, Hameentie 57, 00550 Helsinki 55, and †National Board of Health, Helsinki, Finland

Three **Campylobacter jejuni** strains, NCTC 11168, N 104 (bovine origin) and KH 3 (human origin) were inoculated on fresh meat pieces, weighing about 10 g each. The inoculum size varied from $\log_{10}5$ to $\log_{10}6$. The pH of meat pieces varied from 5.80 to 6.20. The inoculated meat pieces were allocated to three treatments: (a) vacuum-packaged; (b) packaged in an atmosphere of 20% CO_2:80% N_2; (c) packaged into sterile petri dishes in anaerobic cultivation boxes, which were filled with a gas mixture of 5% O_2:10% CO_2:85% N_2 (optimal gas atmosphere for the growth of campylobacters). The survival of campylobacter cells was followed at 37 °C for 48 h, at room temperature (20 °C) for 4 days, and at 4 °C for 25 days.

At 37 °C the campylobacter counts of strains NCTC 11168 and N 104 increased in all package treatments during 48 h. At room temperature and at 4 °C the counts of strains NCTC 11168 and N 104 decreased by 1-2 $\log_{10}$ units or 0.5-1 $\log_{10}$ units, respectively, during storage. The survival of the two strains was about similar in all package treatments. The strain KH 3 was most sensitive of the strains studied. At 37 °C its count increased only in the optimal gas atmosphere; at room temperature the strain was not detectable on the samples after 24-48 h storage, and at 4 °C after 4 days storage. The aerobic plate counts were determined from all samples at same times as campylobacter counts. The high intrinsic bacterial numbers of meat samples did not seem to have great effect on the survival or growth of campylobacters.

g each. The inoculum levels ranged from 10^6 to 10^{10} cfu/g [illegible] of meat pieces varied from [illegible]. The inoculated meat pieces were allocated to storage treatments: (a) vacuum-packaged, (b) packaged in an atmosphere of 20% CO_2 and [illegible], (c) packaged into sterile petri dishes (the anaerobic) [illegible] boxes, which were [illegible] within [illegible] [illegible] (Oxoid) [illegible] for the growth of campylobacters. The survival of campylobacter cells was followed [illegible] 48 h, at room temperature (20 °C) for 4 days and at 4 °C for [illegible] days.

At 37 °C the campylobacter counts of strains NCTC 11168 and N [illegible] increased in all package treatments during 48 h. At room temperature and at 4 °C the counts of strains NCTC 11168 and N 104 decreased by [illegible] log units [illegible], respectively, during storage. The survival of the two strains was about similar in all package treatments. The strain [illegible] was most sensitive of the strains studied. At 37 °C its count increased only in the optimal gas atmosphere; at room temperature the strain was not detectable on the samples after 24–48 h storage and at 4 °C after [illegible] days storage. The aerobic plate counts were determined from all samples at same times as campylobacter counts. The high initial bacterial numbers of meat samples did not seem to have great effect on the survival or growth of campylobacters.

Campylobacter jejuni and the Poultry Industry

INTRODUCTION

An informal meeting was convened to discuss the current state of knowledge on campylobacter infections with respect to the poultry industry. A major aim was to take advantage of the assembled expertise in order to provide information that might be useful when deciding priorities in this area. Twenty-seven interested participants attended the session.

PROCEDURE

Participants were given the following task to complete individually:

> **Given the current state of knowledge with respect to campylobacter infections in man, list specific action steps (if any) you would recommend to a poultry producer with campylobacter-positive flocks of chickens.**

A list of 11 recommendations was drawn up and discussed. At the conclusion of this discussion everyone was asked to select what they considered to be the four most important recommendations and assign rank to these items (i.e. the four most important and the least important). Summation of these ranks produced a priority list which was representative of the views of the group. The major recommendations are listed below together with their rankings to give an idea of the consensus on the items. Important features on the discussion of each item are also included.

RECOMMENDATIONS

Recommendation 1 [41 rank votes] Special effort should be made to educate the consumer to ensure that opportunities for cross-contamination from uncooked meat does not occur, and that cooking and refrigeration are adequate.

Presumably campylobacter ccolonisation of poultry poses a similar health risk to salmonellae in birds. No special action needs to be taken with campylobacter; accepted procedures for salmonellae are utterly appropriate. The public needs to be made more aware that uncooked chickens carry these organisms and may pose a threat to health if not handled correctly.

Recommendation 2 [39 rank votes] The elimination of positive flocks and restocking with pathogen-free birds should be considered.

It was accepted that correct husbandry practices make it difficult to ensure campylobacter-free flocks. Also the financial impact of radical changes in procedures would be too great to expect rapid action. However, it was considered that SPF techniques, as developed in the pig industry, could ultimately be an economic proposition.

Recommendation 3 [35 rank votes] Poultry producers and processors should ensure that standard procedures accepted to reduce **Salmonella** colonisation are actively enforced.

Recommendation 4 [29 rank votes] High quality basic training of staff in the principles of good hygiene is essential. Adherence to currently accepted good manufacturing practice will ensure that contamination loading of **Campylobacter jejuni** is reduced.

Once again the feeling of the meeting was, "like salmonellae, we have to live with campylobacters in processed poultry". However, well trained staff, good hygiene and a responsible approach by management will reduce the problem.

RESEARCH PRIORITIES FOR THE POULTRY INDUSTRY

The following areas were identified as being in need of intensive research effort to allow the drafting of more specific recommendations to the industry:

(a) More basic information is required on the epidemiology of campylobacter colonisation of chicken flocks, i.e. where does it come from, the role of wild birds, how is it transmitted, etc.

(b) Evaluation is required of potential ways of disinfecting processed poultry meat, e.g. by air cooling, by gamma irradiation, by holding carcasses at −20 °C for at least 2 weeks, etc.

(c) Better control is necessary of organisms in chiller water (spray cooling).

(d) More evidence must be sought on the frequency of chicken as a source of campylobacter infection and its mode of transmission.

CONCLUSIONS

There is not enough information yet available to justify any specific initiative in either the poultry production industry or the processing industry with respect to campylobacters. However, the feeling of the group was that there is an urgent need for more research initiatives in the areas previously mentioned to try and reduce the problem of both campylobacters and salmonellae in chickens.

A. Lee

School of Microbiology,
University of New South Wales,
Kensington, Australia

A Campylobacter Bibliography, 1981-1983

The following bibliography is a compilation of most of the significant references to campylobacter literature published since the First International Workshop on Campylobacter Infections (in March 1981) or known to be in press at the time of preparation of the present volume. It does not include reference to any of the papers published in the proceedings of the First International Workshop (D. G. Newell (Ed.) (1981). Campylobacter: Epidemiology, Pathogenesis and Biochemistry, PHLS, London).

For the convenience of the reader, the same heading classification has been used in this bibliography as has been used in the preceding contents of this volume (in so far as possible).

M. B. Skirrow

Department of Microbiology (Pathology),
Royal Infirmary, Worcester, UK

GENERAL REVIEWS

Blaser, M J (1982). **Campylobacter jejuni** and food. Food Technology, **1982**, 89-92.

Butzler, J P (Ed.) (1984). Campylobacter Infection in Man and Animals. CRC Press, Boca Raton, in press [all aspects; 30 authors].

Megraud, F, and Latrille, J (1981). **Campylobacter jejuni** en pathologie humaine. I. Aspects cliniques et therapeutiques [**Campylobacter jejuni** in human pathology. I. Clinical and therapeutic aspects]. Pathologie et Biologie, Paris, **29**, 245-253 [English summary].

Megraud, F, and Latrille J (1981). **Campylobacter jejuni** en pathologie humaine. II. Diagnostic biologique et epidemiologie [**Campylobacter jejuni** in human pathology. II. Biological diagnosis and epidemiology]. Pathologie et Biologie, Paris, **29**, 305-314 [English summary].

Skirrow, M B (1982). Campylobacter enteritis - the first five years. Journal of Hygiene, Cambridge, **89**, 175-184 [epidemiology and public health].

Skirrow, M B (1984). Campylobacter infections of man. In: Medical Microbiology, Vol. 4 (C S F Easmon and J Jeljaszewicz, eds). Academic Press, London, in press [mainly clinical].

I. CLINICAL AND THERAPEUTIC ASPECTS

A. CLINICAL ASPECTS

1. Infections due to campylobacters other than C. jejuni and C. coli

Grob, J P, Francioli, P, and Glauser, M P (1982). Septicemia due to **Campylobacter** ssp. **intestinalis** in immunocompromised patients. Experientia, **38**, 1363.

Righter, J, Wells, W A, Hart, G D, and McNeely, D J (1983). Relapsing septicemia caused by **Campylobacter fetus** subsp. **fetus**. Canadian Medical Association Journal, **128**, 686-689.

Suc, Ch, Moatti, N, Vergnes, D, and Botreau, Y (1983). La contribution de l'haemoculture au diagnostic des trois campylobacterioses humaines. Medecine et Maladies Infectieuses, **13**, 322-327.

Ullmann, U, Langmaack, H, and Blasius, Ch (1982). Campylobacteriosis des Munschen durch die Subspezies **intestinalis** und **fetus** unter Beruecksichtigungsechs neuer Erkrankungen [Six new manifestations of human campylobacteriosis caused by subspecies **intestinalis** and **fetus**]. Europaische Zeitschift fur Klinik und Therapie der Infektionen, **10**, 64-66 [English summary].

Warren, J R, and Marshall, B (1983). Unidentified curved bacilli on gastric epithelium in active chronic gastritis. The Lancet, **i**, 1273-1274 [letters].

2. Infections due to C. jejuni and C. coli

Balakrish Nair, G, Bhattacharya, S K, and Pal, S C (1983). Isolation and characterization of **Campylobacter jejuni** from acute diarrhoeal cases in Calcutta. Transactions of the Royal Society of Tropical Medicine and Hygiene, **77**, 474-476.

Blaser, M J, Wells, J G, Feldman, R A, Pollard, R A, Allen, J R, and The Collaborative Diarrheal Disease Study Group, Atlanta, Georgia (1983). Campylobacter enteritis in the United States: a multicenter study. Annals of Internal Medicine, **98**, 360-365.

Chan, F T H, Stringel, G, and Mackenzie, A M R (1983). Isolation of **Campylobacter jejuni** from an appendix. Journal of Clinical Microbiology, **18**, 422-424.

Constant, O C, Bentley, C C, Denman, A M, Lehane, J R, and Larson, H E (1983). The Guillain-Barre syndrome following **Campylobacter** enteritis with recovery after plasmapheresis. Journal of Infection, **6**, 89-91.

De Mol, P, Hemelhof, W, Butzler, J P, Brasseur, D, Kalala, T, and Vis, H L (1983). Enteropathogenic agents in children with diarrhoea in rural Zaire. The Lancet, **i**, 516-518.

Dickgiesser, A (1983). Campylobacter infektion und haemolytisch-uraemisches Syndrom [Campylobacter infection and haemolytic uraemic syndrome]. Immunitat und Infektionen, **11**, 71–74.

Drake, A A, Gilchrist, M J, Washington, J A, II, Huizenga, K A, and Van Scoy, R E (1982). Diarrhea due to **Campylobacter fetus** subsp. **jejuni**: a clinical review of 63 cases. Mayo Clinic Proceedings, **56**, 414–423.

Eastmond, C J, Rennie, J A N, and Reid, T M S (1982). Campylobacter reactive arthritis – an epidemiological study. Annals of the Rheumatic Diseases, **41**, 312.

Ellis, M E, Pope, J, Mokashi, A, and Dunbar, E (1982). Campylobacter colitis associated with erythema nodosum. The British Medical Journal, **ii**, 937.

Guandalini, S, Cucchiara, S, de Ritis, G, Capano, G, Caprioli, A, Falbo, V, Giraldi, V, Guarino, A, Vairano, P, and Rubino, A (1983). Campylobacter colitis in infants. Journal of Pediatrics, **102**, 72–74.

Gilbert, G L, Davoren, R A, Cole, M E, and Radford, N J (1981). Midtrimester abortion associated with septicaemia caused by **Campylobacter jejuni**. The Medical Journal of Australia, **1**, 585–586.

Goodman, L J, Kaplan, R L, Trenholme, G M, Landau, W, and Kwiatkowski-Barrett, J E (1981). **Campylobacter fetus** subsp. **jejuni**: experience in a large Chicago medical centre. The American Journal of the Medical Sciences, **282**, 125–130.

Gribble, M J, Salit, I E, Isaac-Renton, J, and Chow, A W (1981). Campylobacter infections in pregnancy (case report and literature review). American Journal of Obstetrics and Gynecology, **140**, 423–426.

Hoverson, D B, Blaser, M J, Brown, W R, Ely, I G, Duncan, D J, and Wang, W-L L (1982). Studies on the relationship of **Campylobacter jejuni** infection and inflammatory bowel disease. Gastroenterology, **82**, 1087 [abstract].

Jewkes, J, Larson, H E, Price, A B, Sanderson, P J, and Davies, H A (1981). Aetiology of acute diarrhoea in adults. Gut, **22**, 388–392.

Kirubakaran, C, and Davidson, G P (1981). Campylobacter as a cause of acute enteritis in children in South Australia. II. Clinical comparison with salmonella, rotavirus and non-specific enteritis. The Medical Journal of Australia, **1**, 336.

Kist, M, Keller, K-M, Niebling, W, and Kilching, W (1983). **Campylobacter coli** septicaemia associated with septic abortion. Infection, in press.

Lambert, J R, and Newman, A (1982). **Campylobacter jejuni** causing relapse in chronic inflammatory bowel disease. Australia and New Zealand Journal of Medicine, **12**, 112–113.

Lambert, M, Marion, E, Coche, E, and Butzler, J P (1982). Campylobacter enteritis and erythema nodosum. The Lancet, **i**, 1409 [letter].

Lloyd-Evans, N, Drasar, B S, and Tomkins, A M (1983). A comparison of the prevalence of campylobaccter, shigellae and salmonellae in faeces of malnourished and well nourished children in The Gambia and Northern Nigeria. Transactions of the Royal Society for Tropical Medicine and Hygiene, **77**, 245–247.

McKendrick, M W, Geddes, A M, and Gearty, J (1982). Campylobacter enteritis: a study of clinical features and rectal mucosal changes. Scandinavian Journal of Infectious Diseases, **14**, 35-38.

Mandal, B K (1981). Intestinal infections in adults and children over the age of two. Medicine, **1981**, 56-61.

Melamed, I, Bujanover, Y, Igra, Y S, Schwarz, D, Zakuth, V, and Spirer, Z (1983). **Campylobacter** enteritis in normal and immunodeficient children. American Journal of Diseases of Children, **137**, 752-753.

Menck, H (1981). **Campylobacter jejuni** enteritis kompliceret met glomerulonephritis [**Campylobacter jejuni** enteritis complicated by glomerulonephritis]. Ugeskrift for Laeger, **143**, 1020-1021 [English summary].

Muytjens, H L, and Hoogenhout, J (1982). **Campylobacter jejuni** isolated from a chest wall abscess. Clinical Microbiology Newsletter, **1982**, **166**.

Nayyar, S, Bhan, M K, Gupta, U, Arora, N K, Ghai, O P, Mohapatra, L N, Stinzing, G, Molby, R, and Holme, T (1983). **Campylobacter jejuni** as a cause of childhood diarrhoea in a North Indian community. Journal of Diarrhoeal Diseases Research, **1**, 26-28.

Olarte, J, and Perez, G I (1983). **Campylobacter jejuni** in children with diarrhea in Mexico City. Pediatric Infectious Disease, **2**, 18-20.

Pearce, C T (1981). **Campylobacter jejuni** infection as a cause of septic abortion. Australian Journal of Medical Laboratory Science, **2**, 107-110.

Piemont, Y (1983). Intestinal occurrence of **Campylobacter jejuni** in a French hospitalized population. European Journal of Clinical Microbiology, **2**, 150-152.

Pitkanen, T, Pettersson, T, Ponka, A, and Kosunen, T U (1981). Clinical and serological studies in patients with **Campylobacter fetus** ssp. **jejuni** infection. I. Clinical findings. Infection, **9**, 274-278.

Pitkanen, T, Ponka, A, Pettersson, T, and Kosunen, T U (1983). **Campylobacter** enteritis in 188 hospitalized patients. Archives of Internal Medicine, **143**, 215-218.

Quinn, T C, Stamm, W E, Goodell, S E, Mkrtichian, P A, Benedetti, J, Corey, L, Schuffler, M D, and Holmes, K K (1983). The polymicrobial origin of intestinal infections in homosexual men. New England Journal of Medicine, **309**, 576-582.

Reddy, K R, and Thomas, E (1982). **Campylobacter jejuni** enterocolitis and hepatitis. Gastroenterology, **82**, 1156 [abstract].

Rhodes, K M, and Tattersfield, A E (1982). Guillain-Barre syndrome associated with campylobacter infection. British Medical Journal, **285**, 173-174.

Richardson, N J, Koornhof, H J, and Bokkenheuser, V D (1981). Long-term infections with **Campylobacter fetus** subsp. **jejuni**. Journal of Clinical Microbiology, **13**, 846-849.

Richardson, N J, Koornhoff, H J, Bokkenheuser, V D, Mayet, Z, and Rosen, E U (1983). Age related susceptibility to **Campylobacter jejuni** infection in a high prevalence population. Archives of Diseases in Childhood, **58**, 616-619.

Robinson, D A (1981). Infective dose of **Campylobacter jejuni** in milk. British Medical Journal, **282**, 1584.

Rusu, V, Paigu, L, Dorobat, O, and Zaharia, V (1982). Evaluation of **Campylobacter jejuni** incidence in enteritis; biologic characteristics of isolated strains. Archives Roumaine de Pathologie Experimentalle et Microbiologie, **41**, 303-309.

Schaad, U B (1982). Reactive arthritis associated with campylobacter enteritis. Pediatric Infectious Disease, **1**, 328-332.

Schwartz, R H, Bryan, C, Rodriguez, W J, Park, C, and McCoy, P (1983). Experience with the microbiologic diagnosis of campylobacter enteritis in an office laboratory. Pediatric Infectious Diseases, **2**, 298-301.

Shucheng, D, Shunlin, W, Weiyu, L, Huilan, S, and Weizhong, G (1983). Campylobacter enteritis in infants and young children in China. Journal of Diarrhoeal Diseases Research, **1**, 17-19.

Stoll, B J, Glass, R I, Huq, M I, Khan, M U, Holt, J E, and Banu, H (1982). Surveillance of patients attending a diarrhoeal disease hospital in Bangladesh. British Medical Journal, **285**, 1185-1188.

Sumathipala, R W, and Morrison, G W (1983). Campylobacter enteritis after falling into sewage. British Medical Journal, **286**, 1356 [letter].

Svedhem, A, Kaijser, B, and MacDowell, I (1982). Intestinal occurrence of **Campylobacter fetus** subsp. **jejuni** and **Clostridium difficile** in children in Sweden. European Journal of Clinical Microbiology, **1**, 29-32.

Thoren, A, Stintzing, G, Tufvesson, B, Walder, M, and Habte, D (1982). Aetiology and clinical features of severe infantile diarrhoea in Addis Ababa, Ethiopia. Journal of Tropical Pediatrics, **28**, 127-131.

Vernon, S E, and Dominguez, C (1982). Campylobacter and peritoneal dialysis. Annals of Internal Medicine, **96**, 534 [letter].

Wright, E P (1983). Attempts to isolate **Campylobacter jejuni** from various body sites. Journal of Clinical Pathology, **36**, 667-669.

Wright, E P, Balsdon, M J, and Okubadejo, O A (1982). Isolation of **Campylobacter jejuni** from cervix. The Lancet, **ii**, 380 [letter].

B. THERAPEUTIC ASPECTS

1. Antimicrobial sensitivities and sensitivity testing

Al-Mashat, R R, and Taylor, D J (1983). In vitro sensitivity of 28 bovine isolates of campylobacter to some commonly used antimicrobials. Veterinary Record, **113**, 89.

Anders, B J, Lauer, B A, Paisley, J W, and Reller, L B (1982). Double-blind placebo controlled trial of erythromycin for treatment of campylobacter enteritis. The Lancet, **i**, 131-132.

Buck, G E, and Kelly, M T (1982). Susceptibility testing of **Campylobacter**

fetus subsp. **jejuni** using broth microdilution panels. Antimicrobial Agents and Chemotherapy, **21**, 274-277.

Hof, H, Sticht-Groh, V, and Muller, K-M (1982). Comparative in vitro activities of niridazole and metronidazole against anaerobic and microaerophilic bacteria. Antimicrobial Agents and Chemotherapy, **22**, 332-333.

Michel, J, Rogol, M, and Dickman, D (1983). Susceptibility of clinical isolates of **Campylobacter jejuni** to sixteen antimicrobial agents. Antimicrobial Agents and Chemotherapy, **23**, 796-797.

Primavesi, C A (1983). Untersuchungen zur Antibiotikaempfindlichkeit von **Campylobacter jejuni** [Examinations of the antibiotic sensitivity of **Campylobacter jejuni**]. Hygiene und Medizin, **8**, 138-140 [English summary].

Spelhaug, D R, Gilchrist, M J R, and Washington, J A, II (1981). Bactericidal activity of antibiotics against **Campylobacter fetus** subsp. **intestinalis**. Journal of Infectious Diseases, **143**, 500.

Svedhem, A, Kaijser, B, and Sjogren, E (1981). Antimicrobial susceptibility of **Campylobacter jejuni** isolated from humans with diarrhoea and from healthy chickens. Journal of Antimicrobial Chemotherapy, **7**, 301-305.

Vanhoof, R, Goossens, H, Coignau, H, Stas, G, and Butzler, J P (1982). Susceptibility pattern of **Campylobacter jejuni** from human and animal origins to different antimicrobial agents. Antimicrobial Agents and Chemotherapy, **21**, 990-992.

Welkos, S L (1982). A modified broth-disk antibiotic susceptibility test for **Campylobacter jejuni**. European Journal of Clinical Microbiology, **1**, 354-360.

2. Therapy and clinical trials

Gellert, M, Nyerges, G, Pinter, M, Ban, E, and Bognar, S (1982). Erythromycin therapy in infants' **Campylobacter jejuni** enteritis: a controlled study. In Abstracts of the VIIIth International Congress on Infectious Parasitological Diseases, Stockholm, 1982, p. 70 [abstract].

Pai, C H, Gillis, F, Tuomanen, E, and Marks, M I (1983). Erythromycin in treatment of **Campylobacter** enteritis in children. American Journal of Diseases of Children, **137**, 286-288.

Pitkanen, T, Pettersson, T, Ponka, A, and Kosunen, T U (1982). Effect of erythromycin on the fecal excretion of **Campylobacter fetus** subsp. **jejuni**. Journal of Infectious Diseases, **145**, 128.

Robins-Browne, R M, Mackenjee, M K R, Bodasing, M N, and Coovadia, H M (1983). Treatment of **Campylobacter**-associated enteritis with erythromycin. American Journal of Diseases of Children, **137**, 282-285.

3. Plasmids

Ambrosio, R E, and Lastovica, A J (1983). Rapid screening procedure for detection of plasmids in **Campylobacter**. South African Journal of Science, **79**, 110-111.

Bradbury, W C, Marko, M A, Hennessy, J N, and Penner, J L (1983). Occurrence of plasmid DNA in serologically defined strains of **Campylobacter jejuni** and **Campylobacter coli**. Infection and Immunity, **40**, 460-463.

Taylor, D E, De Grandis, S A, Karmali, M A, and Fleming, P C (1981). Transmissable plasmids from **Campylobacter jejuni**. Antimicrobial Agents and Chemotherapy, **19**, 831-835.

Taylor, D E, Newell, D G, and Pearson, A D (1983). Incidence of plasmid DNA in strains of **Campylobacter jejuni** isolated from stool specimens at 37 °C and 43 °C. Journal of Infectious Diseases, **83**, 965-966 [letter].

Tenover, F C, Brondson, M A, Gordon, K P, and Plorde, J J (1983). Isolation of plasmids encoding tetracycline resistance for **Campylobacter jejuni** strains isolated from simians. Antimicrobial Agents and Chemotherapy, **23**, 320-322.

II. TAXONOMY, BIOTYPING, ISOLATION AND DETECTION

A. TAXONOMY AND BIOTYPING

Skerman, V B D, McGowan, V, and Sneath, P H A (1980). Approved lists of bacterial names. International Journal of Systematic Bacteriology, **30**, 225, 270-271.

1. Molecular aspects

Belland, R J, and Trust, T J (1982). Deoxyribonucleic acid sequence relatedness between thermophilic members of the genus **Campylobacter**. Journal of General Microbiology, **128**, 2515-2522.

Curtis, M A (1983). Cellular fatty acid profiles of campylobacters. Medical Laboratory Sciences, **40**, 333-348.

Hanna, J, Neill, S D, O'Brien, J J, and Ellis, W A (1983). Comparison of aerotolerant and reference strains of campylobacter species by polyacrylamide gel electrophoresis. International Journal of Systematic Bacteriology, **33**, 143-146.

Harvey, S M, and Greenwood, J R (1983). Relationships among catalase-positive campylobacters determined by deoxyribonucleic acid-deoxyribonucleic acid hybridization. International Journal of Systematic Bacteriology, **33**, 275-284.

Leaper, S, and Owen, R J (1981). Identification of catalase-producing **Campylobacter** species based on biochemical characteristics and on cellular fatty acid composition. Current Microbiology, **6**, 31-35.

Leaper, S, and Owen, R J (1982). Differentiation between **Campylobacter jejuni** and allied thermophilic campylobacters by hybridization of deoxyribonucleic acids. FEMS Microbiology Letters, **15**, 203-208.

Owen R J (1983). Nucleic acids in the classification of campylobacters. European Journal of Clinical Microbiology, **2**, 367-377.

Owen, R J, and Leaper, S (1981). Base composition, size and nucleotide sequence similarities of genome deoxyribonucleic acids from species of the genus **Campylobacter**. FEMS Microbiology Letters, **12**, 395-400.

Ursing, J, Walder, M, and Sandstedt, K (1983). Base composition and sequence homology of deoxyribonucleic acid of thermotolerant **Campylobacter** from human and animal sources. Current Microbiology, **8**, 307-310.

2. Biotyping (mainly **C. jejuni**, **C. coli** and **C. laridis**)

Doyle, M P, and Roman, D J (1982). Response of **Campylobacter jejuni** to sodium chloride. Applied and Environmental Microbiology, **43**, 561-565.

Hebert, G A, Hollis, D G, Weaver, R E, Lambert, M A, Blaser, M J, and Moss, C W (1982). 30 years of campylobacters: biochemical characteristics and a biotyping proposal for **Campylobacter jejuni**. Journal of Clinical Microbiology, **15**, 1065-1073.

Hollander, R (1982). Biotyping of **Campylobacter jejuni/coli** isolates from human and animal specimens. Zentralblatt fur Bakteriologie und Hygiene, I. Abteilung Originale A, **251**, 450 [abstract].

Luechtefeld, N W, and Wang, W-L L (1982). Hippurate hydrolysis by and triphenyltetrazolium tolerance of **Campylobacter fetus**. Journal of Clinical Microbiology, **15**, 137-140.

Razi, M H H, Park, R W A, and Skirrow, M B (1981). Two new tests for differentiating between strains of **Campylobacter**. Journal of Applied Bacteriology, **50**, 55-57.

Veron, M, Lenvoise-Furet, A, and Beaune, P (1981). Anaerobic respiration of fumarate as a differential test between **Campylobacter fetus** and **Campylobacter jejuni**. Current Microbiology, **6**, 349-354.

Walder, M, Sandstedt, K, and Ursing, J (1983). Phenotypical characteristics of thermotolerant **Campylobacter** from human and animal sources. Current Microbiology, in press.

3. Morphological aspects

Buck, G E, Parshall, K A, and Davis, C P (1983). Electron microscopy of the coccoid form of **Campylobacter jejuni**. Journal of Clinical Microbiology, **18**, 420-421.

Karmali, M A, Allen, A K, and Fleming, P C (1981). Differentiation of catalase-positive campylobacters with special reference to morphology. International Journal of Systematic Bacteriology, **31**, 64-71.

Kodaka, H, Armfield, A Y, Lombard, G L, and Dowell, V R (1982). Practical procedure for demonstrating bacterial flagella. Journal of Clinical Microbiology, **16**, 948-952.

Lai, C-H, Listgarten, M A, Tanner, A C R, and Socransky, S S (1981). Ultrastructures of **Bacteroides gracilis**, **Campylobacter concisus**, **Wolinella recta** and **Eikenella corrodens**, all from humans with periodontal disease. International Journal of Systematic Bacteriology, **31**, 465-475.

Morooka, T, Umeda, A, and Amako, K (1982). Morphological differences between **Campylobacter jejuni** and **C. fetus.** Japanese Journal of Bacteriology, **37**, 939-941.

4. Newly described campylobacter-like organisms

Badger, S J, and Tanner, A C R (1981). Serological studies of **Bacteroides gracilis, Campylobacter concisus, Wolinella recta** and **Eikenella corrodens,** all from humans with periodontal disease. International Journal of Systematic Bacteriology, **31**, 446-451.

Benjamin, J, Leaper, S, Owen, R J, and Skirrow, M B (1983). Description of **Campylobacter laridis**, a new species comprising the nalidixic acid resistant thermophilic **Campylobacter** (NARTC) group. Current Microbiology, **8**, 231-238.

Gebhart, C J, Ward, G E, Chang, K, and Kurtz, H J (1983). **Campylobacter hyointestinalis** (new species) isolated from swine with lesions of proliferative ileitis. American Journal of Veterinary Research, **44**, 361-367.

Lawson, G H K, Leaver, J L, Pettigrew, G W, and Rowland, A C (1981). Some features of **Campylobacter sputorum** subsp. **mucosalis** subsp. nov., nom. rev., and their taxonomic significance. International Journal of Systematic Bacteriology, **31**, 385-391.

Sandstedt, K, Ursing, J, and Walder, M (1983). Thermotolerant **Campylobacter** with no or weak catalase activity isolated from dogs. Current Microbiology, **8**, 209-213.

Tanner, A C R, Badger, S, Lai, C-H, Listgarten, M A, Visconti, R A, and Socransky, S S (1981). **Wolinella** gen. nov., **Wolinella succinogenes (Vibrio succinogenes** Wolin **et al.**) comb. nov., and description of **Bacteriodes gracilis** sp. nov., **Wolinella recta** sp. nov., **Campylobacter concisus** sp. nov. and **Eikenella corrodens** from humans with periodontal disease. International Journal of Systematic Bacteriology, **31**, 432-445.

B. ISOLATION AND DETECTION

1. Detection by microscopy

Ho, D D, Ault, M J, Ault, M A, and Murata, G H (1982). Campylobacter enteritis: early diagnosis with Gram's stain. Archives of Internal Medicine, **142**, 1858.

Park, C H, Hixon, D L, Polhemus, A S, Ferguson, C B, Hall, S L, Risheim, C C, and Cook, C B (1983). A rapid diagnosis of **Campylobacter** enteritis by direct smear examination. American Journal of Clinical Pathology, **80**, 388-390.

Sazie, E S M, and Titus, A E (1982). Rapid diagnosis of campylobacter enteritis. Annals of Internal Medicine, **96**, 62-63.

2. Transport and preservation

Balakrish Nair, G, and Pal, S C (1982). Short-term preservation medium for **Campylobacter fetus** subspecies **jejuni**. Indian Journal of Medical Research, **76**, 692-695.

Luechtefeld, N W, Wang, W-L L, Blaser, M J, and Reller, L B (1981). Evaluation of transport and storage techniques for isolation of **Campylobacter fetus** subsp. **jejuni** from turkey cecal specimens. Journal of Clinical Microbiology, **13**, 438-443.

Quinn, P J, and Gilchrist, J R (1982). A comparison of transport systems for the recovery of **Campylobacter fetus** ssp. **jejuni**. In Abstracts of the Annual Meeting of the American Society of Microbiology, American Society of Microbiology, Washington, DC, p. 298 [abstract].

Ullman, U, and Kischkel, S (1981). Survival of **Campylobacter** species. Infection, **9**, 210 [letter].

3. Culture media and methods

Acuff, G R, Vanderzant, C, Gardner, F A, and Golan, F A (1982). Evaluation of an enrichment plating procedure for the recovery of **Campylobacter jejuni** from turkey eggs and meat. Journal of Food Protection, **45**, 1276-1278.

Bolton, F J, and Coates, D (1983). Development of a blood-free **Campylobacter** medium: screening tests on basal media and supplements, and the ability of selected supplements to facilitate aerotolerance. Journal of Applied Bacteriology, **54**, 115-125.

Bolton, F J, and Robertson, L (1982). A selective medium for isolating **Campylobacter jejuni/coli**. Journal of Clinical Pathology, **35**, 462-467.

Bolton, F J, Coates, D, Hinchliffe, P M, and Robertson, L (1983). Comparison of selective media for isolation of **Campylobacter jejuni/coli**. Journal of Clinical Pathology, **36**, 78-83.

Bolton, F J, Hutchinson, D N, and Coates, D (1983). A blood-free selective medium for the isolation of **Campylobacter jejuni** from faeces. Journal of Clinical Microbiology, in press.

Bopp, C A, Wells, J G, and Barrett, T J (1982). Trimethoprim activity in media selective for **Campylobacter jejuni**. Journal of Clinical Microbiology, **16**, 808-812.

Buck, G E, and Kelly, M T (1981). Effect of moisture content of the medium on colony morphology of **Campylobacter fetus** subsp. **jejuni**. Journal of Clinical Microbiology, **14**, 585-586.

Butzler, J P, De Boeck, M, and Goossens, H (1983). New selective medium for isolation of **Campylobacter jejuni** from faecal specimens. The Lancet, **i**, in press.

Chan, F T H, and Mackenzie, A M R (1983). Advantage of using enrichment culture techniques to isolate **Campylobacter jejuni** from stools. Journal of Infectious Diseases, in press.

Doyle, M P, and Roman, D J (1982). Recovery of **Campylobacter jejuni** and

Campylobacter coli from inoculated foods by selective enrichment. Applied and Environmental Microbiology, **43**, 1343-1353.

Garcia, M M, Ruckerbauer, G M, Eaglesome, M D, and Boisclair, W E (1983). Detection of **Campylobacter fetus** in artificial insemination bulls with a transport enrichment medium. Canadian Journal of Comparative Medicine, **47**, 336-340.

Gilchrist, M J R, Grewell, C M, and Washington, J A, II (1981). Evaluation of media for isolation of **Campylobacter fetus** subsp. **jejuni** from fecal specimens. Journal of Clinical Microbiology, **14**, 393-395.

Goossens, H, de Boeck, M, and Butzler, J P (1983). A new selective medium for the isolation of **Campylobacter jejuni** from human faeces. European Journal of Clinical Microbiology, **2**, 389-393.

Hanninen, M-L (1982). Comparison of four enrichment media in the recovery of **Campylobacter jejuni**. Acta Veterinaria Scandinavica, **23**, 425-437.

Janssen, D, and Helstad, A G (1982). Isolation of **Campylobacter fetus** subsp. **jejuni** from human fecal specimens by incubation at 35 and 42 °C. Journal of Clinical Microbiology, **16**, 398-399.

Lovett, J, Francis, D W, and Hunt, J (1982). A method for isolating **Campylobacter fetus** subsp. **jejuni** from raw milk. In Abstracts of the Annual Meeting of the American Society of Microbiology, American Society of Microbiology, Washington, DC, p. 209 [abstract].

Martin, W T, Patton, C M, Morris, G K, Potter, M E, and Puhr, N D (1983). Selective enrichment broth medium for isolation of **Campylobacter jejuni**. Journal of Clinical Microbiology, **17**, 853-855.

Moskowitz, L B, and Chester, B (1982). Growth of non-**Campylobacter**, oxidase-positive bacteria on selective **Campylobacter** agar. Journal of Clinical Microbiology, **15**, 1144-1147.

Park, C E, Stankiewicz, Z K, Lovett, J, Hunt, J, and Francis, D W (1983). Effect of temperature, duration of incubation, and pH of enrichment culture on the recovery of **Campylobacter jejuni** from eviscerated market chickens. Canadian Journal of Microbiology, **29**, 803-806.

Patton, C M, Mitchell, S W, Potter, M E, and Kaufmann, A F (1981). Comparison of selective media for primary isolation of **Campylobacter fetus** subsp. **jejuni**. Journal of Clinical Microbiology, **13**, 326-330.

Richardson, N J, Koornhof, H J, and Bokkenheuser, V D (1982). Primary isolation of **Campylobacter fetus** subspecies **jejuni**. American Journal of Medical Technology, **48**, 197-199.

Rollins, D M, Coolbaugh, J C, Walker, R J, and Weiss, E (1983). Biphasic culture system for rapid **Campylobacter** cultivation. Applied and Environmental Microbiology, **45**, 284-289.

Skirrow, M B, Benjamin, J, Razi, M H H, and Waterman, S (1982). Isolation, cultivation and identification of **Campylobacter jejuni** and **C. coli**. In Isolation and Identification Methods for Food Poisoning Organisms (J E L Corry, D Roberts and F A Skinner, eds), Academic Press, London, pp. 313-328.

Stern, N J (1981). **Campylobacter fetus** ssp. **jejuni**: recovery methodology and isolation from lamb carcasses. Journal of Food Science, **46**, 660-661, 663.

4. Atmospheric requirements

Bolton, F J, and Coates, D (1983). A study of the oxygen and carbon dioxide requirements of thermophilic campylobacters. Journal of Clinical Pathology, **36**, 829-834.

Buck, G E, Fojtasek, C, Calvert, K, and Kelly, M T (1982). Evaluation of the CampyPak II gas generator system for isolation of **Campylobacter fetus** subsp. **jejuni**. Journal of Clinical Microbiology, **15**, 41-42.

Kaplan, R L, Barrett, J E, and Goodman, L J (1982). A simple method for creating an atmosphere to isolate **Campylobacter fetus** subsp. **jejuni**. In Abstracts of the Annual Meeting of the American Society of Microbiology, American Society of Microbiology, Washington, DC, p. 300 [abstract].

Luechtefeld, N W, Reller, L B, Blaser, M J, and Wang, W-L L (1982). Comparison of atmospheres of incubation for primary isolation of **Campylobacter fetus** subsp. **jejuni** frtom animal specimens: 5% oxygen versus candle jar. Journal of Clinical Microbiology, **15**, 53-57.

Magalhaes, M, and Andrade, M de A (1982). Simple and inexpensive method for culturing **Campylobacter fetus** subsp. **jejuni**. Revista Microbiologia, Sao Paulo, **13**, 124-125.

Reller, L B, Mirrett, S, Paisley, J W, Roe, M, and Lauer, B A (1982). Field trial comparison of atmospheres achieved with CampyPak II and candle jar for clinical isolation of **Campylobacter jejuni** from human fecal specimens. In Abstracts of the Annual Meeting of the American Society of Microbiology, American Society of Microbiology, Washington, DC, p. 299 [abstract].

Wang, W-L L, Luechtefeld, N W, Blaser, M J, and Reller, L B (1982). Comparison of CampyPak II with standard 5% oxygen and candle jars for growth of **Campylobacter jejuni** from human feces. Journal of Clinical Microbiology, **16**, 291-294.

Wang, W-L L, Luechtefeld, N W, Blaser, M J, and Reller, L B (1983). Effect of incubation atmosphere and temperature on isolation of **Campylobacter jejuni** from human stools. Canadian Journal of Microbiology, **29**, 468-470.

5. Respiratory physiology

Carlone, G M, and Lascelles, J (1982). Aerobic and anaerobic respiratory systems in **Campylobacter fetus** subsp. **jejuni** grown in atmospheres containing hydrogen. Journal of Bacteriology, **152**, 306-314.

El Kurdi, A B, Leaver, J L, and Pettigrew, G W (1982). The c-type cytochromes of **Campylobacter sputorum** spp. **mucosalis**. FEMS Microbiology Letters, **14**, 177-182.

Fletcher, R D, Albers, A C, Chen, A K, and Albertson, J N (1983). Ascorbic acid inhibition of **Campylobacter jejuni** growth. Applied and Environmental Microbiology, **45**, 792-795.

Goodman, T G, and Hoffman, P S (1982). Hydrogen and formate oxidation in **Campylobacter jejuni**. In Abstracts of the Annual Meeting of the American Society of Microbiology, American Society of Microbiology, Washington, DC, p. 49 [abstract].

Harvey, S, and Lascelles, J (1980). Respiratory systems and cytochromes in **Campylobacter fetus** subsp. **intestinalis**. Journal of Bacteriology, **144**, 917-922.

Niekus, H G D, and Stouthamer, A H (1981). Formate oxidase in glutaraldehyde-treated **Campylobacter sputorum** subspecies **bubulus**. FEMS Microbiology Letters, **11**, 83-87.

III. ANTIGENS AND SERODIAGNOSIS

A. ANTIGENS

1. Surface antigens

Logan, S M, and Trust, T J (1982). Outer membrane characteristics of **Campylobacter jejuni**. Infection and Immunity, **38**, 898-906.

Naess, V, and Hofstad, T (1982). Isolation and chemical composition of lipopolysaccharide from **Campylobacter jejuni**. Acta Pathologica, Microbiologica et Immunologica Scandinavica B, **90**, 135-139.

B. SERODIAGNOSIS

Blaser, M J, Duncan, D J, Osterholm, M T, Istre, G R, and Wang, W-L L (1983). Serologic study of two clusters of infection due to **Campylobacter jejuni**. Journal of Infectious Diseases, **147**, 820-823.

Figura, N, and Rossolini, A (1982). Evaluation of a commercially available "**Campylobacter fetus** subsp. **jejuni**" antigen in the serologic diagnosis of campylobacter enteritis. Bollettino del Istituto Sieroter, Milano, **61**, 520-522 [letter].

Jones, D M, Robinson, D A, and Eldridge, J (1981). Serological studies in two outbreaks of **Campylobacter jejuni** infection. Journal of Hygiene, Cambridge, **87**, 163-170.

Kahlich, R, Kotlar, V, Palecek, A, Fischer, P, and Malek, J (1982). Prispevek k hodnoceni kampylobakteriozy v CSSR [An outbreak of campylobacter enteritis in Czechoslovakia]. Casopis Lekaru Ceskych, **121**, 1452-1456 [English summary].

Kaldor, J, Pritchard, H, Serpell, A, and Metcalf, W (1983). Serum antibodies in campylobacter enteritis. Journal of Clinical Microbiology, **18**, 1-4.

Kosunen, T U, Pitkanen, T, Pettersson, T, and Ponka, A (1981). Clinical and serological studies in patients with **Campylobacter fetus** ssp. **jejuni** infections: II. Serological findings. Infection, **9**, 279-282.

Kosunen, T U, Rautelin, H, Pitkanen, T, Ponka, A, and Pettersson, T (1983). Antibodies against an acid extract from a single campylobacter strain in hospitalized campylobacter patients. Infection, **11**, 189-191.

Rautelin, H, and Kosunen, T U (1983). An acid extract as a common antigen in **Campylobacter coli** and **Campylobacter jejuni** strains. Journal of Clinical Microbiology, **17**, 700-701.

Svedhem, A, Gunnarsson, H, and Kaijser, B (1983). Diffusion-in-gel enzyme-linked immunosorbent assay for routine detection of IgG and IgM antibodies of **Campylobacter jejuni**. Journal of Infectious Diseases, **148**, 82-92.

Ullmann, U (1981). Seroepidemiological studies with **Campylobacter fetus.** Zentralblatt fur Bakteriologie und Hygiene, I. Abteilung Originale A, **250**, 554-556.

Wassmer, P, Karlen, J, Bumbacher, H J, and Gasser, M (1982). Use of the ELISA technique for demonstration of antibodies against **Campylobacter jejuni**. Experientia, **38**, 1375.

Watson, K C, and Kerr, E J C (1982). Comparison of agglutination, complement fixation and immunofluorescence tests in **Campylobacter jejuni** infections. Journal of Hygiene, Cambridge, **88**, 165-171.

IV. SEROTYPING AND PHAGE TYPING: APPLICATION AND INTERPRETATION

A. SEROTYPING

Hebert, G A, Hollis, D G, Weaver, R E, Steigerwalt, A G, McKinney, R M, and Brenner, D J (1983). Serogroups of **Campylobacter jejuni**, **Campylobacter coli** and **Campylobacter fetus** defined by direct immunofluorescence. Journal of Clinical Microbiology, **17**, 529-538.

Karmali, M A, Penner, J L, and Fleming, P C (1983). The serotype and biotype distribution of clinical isolates of **Campylobacter jejuni** and **Campylobacter coli** over a three-year period. Journal of Infectious Diseases, **147**, 243-246.

Kosunen, T U, Danielsson, D, and Kjellander, J (1982). Serology of **Campylobacter fetus** ss. **jejuni**. 2. Serotyping of live bacteria by slide, latex and co-agglutination tests. Acta Pathologica, Microbiologica et Immunologica Scandinavica B, **90**, 191-196.

Lastovica, A J, and Penner, J L (1983). Serotypes of **Campylobacter jejuni** and **Campylobacter coli** in bacteremic, hospitalized children. Journal of Infectious Diseases, **147**, 592.

Lior, H, Woodward, D L, Edgar, J A, Laroche, L J, and Gill, P (1982). Serotyping of **Campylobacter jejuni** by slide agglutination based on heat-labile antigenic factors. Journal of Clinical Microbiology, **15**, 761-768.

McMyne, P M S, Penner, J L, Mathias, R G, Black, W A, and Hennessy, J N (1982). Serotyping of **Campylobacter jejuni** isolated from sporadic cases and outbreaks in British Columbia. Journal of Clinical Microbiology, **16**,

281-285.

Penner, J L, Hennessy, J N, and Congi, R V (1983). Serotyping of **Campylobacter jejuni** and **Campylobacter coli** on the basis of thermostable antigens. European Journal of Clinical Microbiology, **2**, 378-383.

Rogol, M, Sechter, I, Braunstein, I, and Gerichter, C B (1983). Extended scheme for serotyping **Campylobacter jejuni**: results obtained in Israel from 1980 to 1981. Journal of Clinical Microbiology, **18**, 283-286.

B. PHAGE TYPING

Blackwell, C C, Winstanley, F P, and Telfer Brunton, W A (1982). Sensitivity of thermophilic campylobacters to R-type pyocines of **Pseudomonas aeruginosa.** Journal of Medical Microbiology, **15**, 247-251.

Ritchie, A E, Bryner, J H, and Foley, J W (1983). Role of DNA and bacteriophage in campylobacter autoagglutination. Journal of Medical Microbiology, **16**, 333-340.

V. PATHOGENESIS

D. NATURAL AND EXPERIMENTAL C. JEJUNI INFECTION IN ANIMALS

1. Laboratory rodents

Blaser, M J, Duncan, D J, Warren, G H, and Wang, W-L L (1982). Experimental **Campylobacter jejuni** infection of adult mice. Infection and Immunity, **39**, 908-916.

Field, L H, Underwood, J L, Pope, L M, and Berry, L J (1981). Intestinal colonization of neonatal animals by **Campylobacter fetus** subsp. **jejuni**. Infection and Immunity, **33**, 884-892.

Fox, J G, Zanotti, S, and Jordon, H V (1982). Implantation and distribution of **Campylobacter fetus** subsp. **jejuni** in hamsters. Laboratory Animal Science, **32**, 442.

Kee Peng Ng, F, Wardlaw, A C, and Stewart-Tull, D E S (1980). Enhancement of the lethal effect of **Campylobacter fetus** subsp. **jejuni** in seven-day old mice by ferric ammonium citrate. Society for General Microbiology Quarterly, **8**, 12.

La Regina, M, and Lonigro, J (1982). Isolation of **Campylobacter fetus** subspecies **jejuni** from hamsters with proliferative ileitis. Laboratory Animal Science, **32**, 660-662.

Lentsch, R H, McLaughlin, R M, Wagner, J E, and Day, T J (1982). **Campylobacter fetus** subspecies **jejuni** isolated from Syrian hamsters with proliferative ileitis. Laboratory Animal Science, **32**, 511-514.

Madge, D S (1980). Campylobacter enteritis in young mice. Digestion, **20**, 389-394.

Newell, D G, and Pearson, A D (1983). Invasion of epithelial cell lines and infant mice gastrointestinal epithelium by **C. jejuni/coli**. Journal of Diarrhoeal Disease Research, **1**, in press.

Vandenberghe, J, and Marsboom, R (1982). Campylobacter-like bacteria in adenocarcinomas of the colon in two Wistar rats. Veterinary Record, **111** 416-417.

2. Poultry

Ruiz-Palacios, G M, Escamilla, E, and Torres, N (1981). Experimental campylobacter diarrhea in chickens. Infection and Immunity, **34**, 250-255.

Soerjadi, A S, Snoeyenbos, G H, and Weinack, O M (1982). Intestinal colonization and competitive exclusion of **Campylobacter fetus** subsp. **jejuni** in young chicks. Avian Diseases, **26**, 520-524.

3. Dogs and cats

McOrist, S, and Browning, J W (1982). Carriage of **Campylobacter jejuni** in healthy and diarrhoeic dogs and cats. Australian Veterinary Journal, **58**, 33-34.

Prescott, J F, Barker, I K, Manninen, K I, and Miniats, O P (1981). **Campylobacter jejuni** colitis in gnotobiotic dogs. Canadian Journal of Comparative Medicine, **45**, 377-383.

Sandstedt, K, and Wierup, M (1980/81). Concomitant occurrence of **Campylobacter** and parvoviruses in dogs with gastroenteritis. Veterinary Research Communications, **4**, 271-273.

Simpson, J W, Burnie, A G, Ferguson, S, and Telfer Brunton, W A (1981). Isolation of thermophilic campylobacters from two populations of dogs. Veterinary Research Communications, **5**, 63-66.

Skirrow, M B (1981). Campylobacter enteritis in dogs and cats: a "new" zoonosis. Veterinary Research Communications, **5**, 13-19.

Vandenberghe, J, Lauwers, S, Plehier, P, and Hoorens, J (1982). **Campylobacter jejuni** related with diarrhoea in dogs. British Veterinary Journal, **138**, 356-361.

4. Monkeys

Bryant, J L, Stills, H F, Lentsch, R H, and Middleton, C C (1983). **Campylobacter jejuni** isolated from Patas monkeys with diarrhea. Laboratory Animal Science, **33**, 303-305.

Fitzgeorge, R B, Baskerville, A, and Lander, K P (1981). Experimental infection of Rhesus monkeys with a human strain of **Campylobacter jejuni**. Journal of Hygiene, Cambridge, **86**, 343-351.

Morton, W R, Bronsdon, M, Mickelsen, G, Knitter, G, Rosenkranz, S, Kuller, La R, and Sajuthi, D (1983). Identification of **Campylobaccter jejuni** in **Macaca fascicularis** imported from Indonesia. Laboratory Animal Science, **33**, 187-188.

Tribe, G W, and Fleming, M P (1983). Biphasic enteritis in imported Cynomolgus (**Macaca fascicularis**) monkeys infected with shigella, salmonella and campylobacter species. Laboratory Animals, **17**, 65-69.

5. Other domestic animals

Al-Mashat, R R, and Taylor, D J (1983). Production of enteritis in calves by the oral inoculation of pure cultures of **Campylobacter fetus** subspecies **intestinalis**. Veterinary Record, **112**, 54-58.

Firehammer, B D, and Myers, L L (1981). **Campylobacter fetus** subsp. **jejuni**: its possible significance in enteric disease of calves and lambs. American Journal of Veterinary Research, **42**, 918-922.

Fox, J G, Newcomer, C E, and Ackerman, J I (1982). **Campylobacter fetus** ss. **jejuni** infection in ferrets: clinical and therapeutic indices. Laboratory Animal Science, **32**, 430 [abstract].

Olubunmi, P A, and Taylor, D J (1982). Production of enteritis in pigs by the oral inoculation of pure cultures of **Campylobacter coli**. Veterinary Record, **111**, 197-202.

Taylor, D J, and Olubumni, P A (1981). A re-examination of the role of **Campylobacter fetus** subspecies **coli** in enteric disease of the pig. Veterinary Record, **109**, 112-115.

Vandenberghe, J, and Hoorens, J (1980). Campylobacter species and regional enteritis in lambs. Research in Veterinary Science, **29**, 390-391.

E. TOXINS

Blankenship, L C, Craven, S E, and Hopkins, S R (1982). Preliminary characterization of a factor(s) from cell extracts of **Campylobacter fetus** subsp. **jejuni** that produces cytotoxic effects in cell cultures. In Abstracts of the Annual Meeting of the American Society of Microbiology, American Society for Microbiology, Washington, DC, p. 205 [abstract].

Fernandez, H, Neto, U F, Fernandes, F, Pedra, M de A, and Trabulsi, L R (1983). Culture supernatants of **Campylobacter jejuni** induce a secretory response in jejunal segments of adult rats. Infection and Immunity, **40**, 429-431.

Manninen, K I, Prescott, J F, and Dohoo, I R (1982). Pathogenicity of **Campylobacter jejuni** isolates from animals and humans. Infection and Immunity, **38**, 46-52.

Ruiz-Palacios, G M, Torres, J, Torres, N I, Escamilla, E, Ruiz-Palacios, B R, and Tamayo, J (1983). Cholera-like enterotoxin produced by **Campylobacter jejuni**: characterization and clinical significance. The Lancet, **i**, 250-254.

Sninsky, C A, Ramphal, R, Gaskins, D J, Martin, J L, Goldberg, D L, and Mathias, J R (1982). **Campylobacter jejuni** or its cell-free filtrate causes altered myoelectric activity. Gastroenterology, **82**, 1184 [abstract].

F. MISCELLANEOUS INFECTIONS

Al-Mashat, R R, and Taylor, D J (1981). Production of enteritis in calves by the oral inoculation of pure cultures of **Campylobacter fecalis.** Veterinary Record, **109**, 97-101.

Anderson, K L, Hamoud, M M, Urbance, J W, Rhoades, M S, and Bryner, J H (1983). Isolation of **Campylobacter jejuni** from an aborted caprine fetus. Journal of the American Veterinary Medicine Association, **183**, 90-92.

Gill, K P W (1983). Aerotolerant campylobacter strain isolated from a bovine preputial sheath washing. Veterinary Record, **112**, 459.

Howard, T H, Vasquez, L A, and Amann, R P (1982). Antibiotic control of **Campylobacter fetus** by three extenders of bovine semen. Journal of Dairy Science, **65**, 1596-1600.

Lawson, G H K, Roberts, L, McCartney, E, Rowland, A C, and Luckins, A G (1982). Presence of serum agglutinins to **Campylobacter sputorum** subspecies **mucosalis** in pigs. Research in Veterinary Science, **32**, 89-94.

Logan, E F, Neill, S D, and Mackie, D P (1982). Mastitis in dairy cows associated with an aerotolerant campylobacter. Veterinary Record, **110**, 229-230.

Mustafa, A A (1981). **Campylobacter fetus** subspecies **intestinalis** in Syria. Veterinary Record, **109**, 515-516.

Neill, S D, Mackie, D P, and Logan, E F (1982). Campylobacter mastitis in dairy cows. Veterinary Record, **110**, 505-506 [letter].

VI. EPIDEMIOLOGY AND SURVIVAL EXPERIMENTS

A. EPIDEMIOLOGY

2. Outbreak studies

Blaser, M J, Checko, P, Bopp, C, and Hughes, J M (1981). Foodborne campylobacter enteritis at a summer camp in Connecticut. In Abstracts of Papers: 30th Annual Conference of the Epidemic Intelligence Service, Centers for Disease Control, Atlanta, Ga, unnumbered [abstract].

Christenson, B, Ringner, A, Blucher, C, Billaudelle, H, Gundtoft, K N, Eriksson, G, and Bottiger, M (1983). An outbreak of campylobacter enteritis among the staff of a poultry abattoir in Sweden. Scandinavian Journal of Infectious Disease, **15**, 167-172.

Goodman, L J, Harris, A A, Sokalski, S J, Kellie, S, Barrett, J E, Ruthe, A, Finn, A, and Kaplan, R L (1983). A restaurant associated campylobacter outbreak. European Journal of Clinical Microbiology, **2**, 394-395 [letter].

Jones, P H, Willis, A T, Robinson, D A, Skirrow, M B, and Josephs, D S (1981). Campylobacter enteritis associated with the consumption of free school milk. Journal of Hygiene, Cambridge, **87**, 155-162.

Kirubakaran, C, Davidson, G P, Darby, H, Hansman, D, McKay, G, Moore, B, and Lee, P (1981). Campylobacter as a cause of acute enteritis in children in South Australia. I. A 12-month study with controls. Medical Journal of Australia, **1**, 333-335.

Kornblatt, A N (1982). Campylobacter enteritis associated with raw milk, Kansas. In Abstracts of Papers: 31st Annual Conference of the Epidemic Intelligence Service, Centers for Disease Control, Atlanta, Ga, pp. 30-31 [abstract].

Mentzing, L-O (1981). Waterborne outbreak of campylobacter enteritis in central Sweden. The Lancet, **ii**, 352.

Osterholm, M, Korlath, J, McCullough, J, and Judy, L (1982). An outbreak of campylobacteriosis associated with uspasteurised milk consumption. American Journal of Epidemiology, **116**, 557 [abstract].

Palmer, S R, Gully, P R, White, J M, Pearson, A D, Suckling, W G, Jones, D M, Rawes, J C L, and Penner, J L (1983). Water-borne outbreak of campylobacter gastroenteritis. The Lancet, **i**, 287-290.

Shandera, W X (1981). Campylobacter septicemia associated with processed turkey. In Abstracts of Papers: 30th Annual Conference of the Epidemic Intelligence Service, Centers for Disease Control, Atlanta, Ga, unnumbered [abstract].

Skirrow, M B, Fidoe, R G, and Jones, D M (1981). An outbreak of presumptive foodborne campylobacter enteritis. Journal of Infection, **3**, 234-236.

Taylor, D N, Porter, B W, William, C A, Miller, H G, Bopp, C A, and Blake, P A (1982). **Campylobacter** enteritis: a large outbreak traced to commercial raw milk. Western Journal of Medicine, **137**, 365-369.

Vogt, R L, Sours, H E, Barrett, T, Feldman, R A, Dickinson, R J, and Witherell, L (1982). Campylobacter enteritis associated with contaminated water. Annals of Internal Medicine, **96**, 292-296.

3. General surveys

Cameron, S, Roder, D, and White, C (1982). Population-based comparative study of campylobacter and salmonella enteritis in South Australia. Medical Journal of Australia, **2**, 175-177.

Dilworth, C R (1983). Campylobacter enteritis: incidence in central New Brunswick, Canada. Canadian Journal of Public Health, **74**, 195-198.

Kalman, M, Nagy, E, Kiss, I, and Horvath, M (1982). **Campylobacter jejuni** enteritis: incidence, age distribution and clinical symptoms. Acta Microbiologica Academiae Scientiarum Hungaricae, **29**, 217-219.

Kendall, E J C, and Tanner, E I (1982). Campylobacter enteritis in general practice. Journal of Hygiene, Cambridge, **88**, 155-163.

Kist, M. (1982). Campylobacter enteritis: frequency, sources and routes of infection. Zentralblatt fur Bakteriologie und Hygiene. I. Abteilung Originale A, **251**, 457 [abstract].

Pien, F D, Hsu, A K, Padua, S A, Isaacson, N S, and Naka, S (1983). **Campylobacter jejuni** enteritis in Honolulu, Hawaii. Transactions of the

Royal Society of Tropical Medicine and Hygiene, **77**, 492-494.

Prasanna Rajan, D, and Mathan, V I (1982). Prevalence of **Campylobacter fetus** subsp. **jejuni** in healthy populations in southern India. Journal of Clinical Microbiology, **15**, 749-751.

Shmilovitz, M, Kretzer, B, and Rotman, N (1982). **Campylobacter jejuni** as an etiological agent of diarrheal diseases in Israel. Israel Journal of Medical Science, **18**, 935-940.

Walder, M (1982). Epidemiology of campylobacter enteritis. Scandinavian Journal of Infectious Diseases, **14**, 27-33.

4. Animal, food and environmental sources

Barot, M S, Mosenthal, A C, and Bokkenheuser, V D (1983). Location of **Campylobacter jejuni** in infected chicken livers. Journal of Clinical Microbiology, **17**, 921-922.

Bolton, F J, Dawkins, H C, and Robertson, L (1982). **Campylobacter jejuni/coli** in abattoirs and butchers shops. Journal of Infection, **4**, 243-245.

Bolton, F J, Hinchliffe, P M, Coates, D, and Robertson, L (1982). A most probable number method for estimating small numbers of campylobacters in water. Journal of Hygiene, Cambridge, **89**, 185-190.

Bruce, D, and Fleming, G A (1983). Campylobacter isolations from household dogs. Veterinary Record, **112**, 16.

Christopher, F M, Smith, G C, and Vanderzant, C (1982). Examination of poultry giblets, raw milk and meat for **Campylobacter fetus** subsp. **jejuni**. Journal of Food Protection, **45**, 260-262.

Echeverria, P, Harrison, B A, Tirapat, C, and McFarland, A (1983). Flies as a source of enteric pathogens in a rural village in Thailand. Applied and Environmental Microbiology, **46**, 32-36.

Elharrif, Z, Megraud, F, Quesnel, J J, and Latrille, J (1982). Sources de **Campylobacter jejuni** [Sources of **Campylobacter jejuni**]. Nouvelle Presse Medicale, **11**, 1419.

Figueroa, G, Troncoso, M, Alcayde, P, and Sepulveda, C (1981). Aislamiento de **Campylobacter fetus** sub-especie **jejuni** en heces de porcinos [Isolation of **Campylobacter fetus** subsp. **jejuni** from faeces of piglets]. Revista Chilena de Technologia Medica, **4**, 6-10.

Figueroa, G, Toledo, S, Troncoso, M, and Sepulveda, C (1982). Aislamiento de **Campylobacter fetus** sub-especie **jejuni** en pollos broiler [Isolation of **Campylobacter fetus** subsp. **jejuni** in broiler chickens]. Revista Chilena de Nutricion, **10**, 87-98.

Fox, J G, Ackerman, J I, and Newcomer, C E (1983). Ferret as a potential reservoir for human campylobacteriosis. American Journal of Veterinary Research, **44**, 1049-1052.

Fox, J G, Zanotti, S, and Jordan, H V (1981). The hamster as a reservoir of **Campylobacter fetus** subspecies **jejuni**. Journal of Infectious Diseases, **143**, 856.

Galbraith, N S, Forbes, P, and Clifford, C (1982). Communicable disease associated with milk and dairy products in England and Wales 1951-80. British Medical Journal, **284**, 1761-1765.

Gill, C O, and Harris, L M (1982). Contamination of red-meat carcasses by **Campylobacter fetus** subsp. **jejuni**. Applied and Environmental Microbiology, **43**, 977-980.

Kapperud, G, and Rosef, O (1983). Avian wildlife reservoir of **Campylobacter fetus** subsp. **jejuni**, **Yersinia** spp. and **Salmonella** spp. in Norway. Applied and Environmental Microbiology, **45**, 375-380.

Kinde, H, Genigeorgis, C A, and Pappiaioanou, M (1983). Prevalence of **Campylobacter jejuni** in chicken wings. Applied and Environmental Microbiology, **45**, 1116-1118.

Lovett, J, Francis, D W, and Hunt, J M (1983). Isolation of **Campylobacter jejuni** from raw milk. Applied and Environmental Microbiology, **46**, 459-462.

Lovett, J, Hunt, J M, and Francis, D W (1982). Survey of fresh market turkey for **Campylobacter jejuni**. Dairy Food Sanitation, **2**, 423 [abstract].

Luechtefeld, N W, and Wang, W-L L (1981). **Campylobacter fetus** subsp. **jejuni** in a turkey processing plant. Journal of Clinical Microbiology, **13**, 266-268.

Luechtefeld, N W, Cambre, R C, and Wang, W-L L (1981). Isolation of **Campylobacter fetus** subsp. **jejuni** from zoo animals. Journal of the American Veterinary Medical Association, **179**, 1119-1122.

Marcola, B, Watkins, J, and Riley, A (1981). The isolation and identification of thermotolerant **Campylobacter** spp. from sewage and river waters. Journal of Applied Bacteriology, **51**, xii-xiv.

Marjai, E, Kovats, Z, Kajary, I, and Horvath, Z (1982). **Campylobacter jejuni** contamination of slaughtered chickens. Acta Microbiologica Academiae Scientiarum Hungaricae, **29**, 213-215.

Oosterom, J, Engels, G B, Peters, R, and Pot, R (1982). **Campylobacter jejuni** in cattle and raw milk in The Netherlands. Journal of Food Protection, **45**, 1212-1213.

Oosterom, J, Notermans, S, Karman, H, and Engels, G B (1983). Origin and prevalence of **Campylobacter jejuni** in poultry processing. Journal of Food Protection, **46**, 339-344.

Oosterom, J, de Wilde, G J A, de Boer, E, de Blaauw, L H, and Karman, H (1983). Survival of **Campylobacter jejuni** during poultry processing and pig slaughtering. Journal of Food Protection, **46**, 702-706, 709.

Ottolenghi, A C, and Hamparian, V V (1982). Bacteriology of sewage sludge; examination for the presence of salmonella and campylobacter. In Abstracts of the Annual Meeting of the American Society of Microbiology, American Society for Microbiology, Washington, DC, p. 214 [abstract].

Park, C E, Stankiewicz, Z K, Lovett, J, and Hunt, J (1981). Incidence of **Campylobacter jejuni** in fresh eviscerated whole market chickens. Canadian

Journal of Microbiology, **27**, 841-842.

Prescott, J F, and Bruin-Mosch, C W (1981). Carriage of **Campylobacter jejuni** in healthy and diarrheic animals. American Journal of Veterinary Research, **42**, 164-165.

Rayes, H M, Genigeorgis, C A, and Farver, T B (1983). Prevalence of **Campylobacter jejuni** on turkey wings at the supermarket level. Journal of Food Protection, **46**, 292-294.

Rosef, O, and Kapperud, G (1983). House flies (**Musca domestica**) as possible vectors of **Campylobacter fetus** subsp. **jejuni**. Applied and Environmental Microbiology, **45**, 381-383.

Shanker, S, Rosenfield, J A, Davey, G R, and Sorrell, T C (1982). **Campylobacter jejuni**: incidence in processed broilers and biotype distribution in human and broiler isolates. Applied and Environmental Microbiology, **43**, 1219-1220.

Smeltzer, T I (1981). Isolation of **Campylobacter jejuni** from poultry carcasses. Australian Veterinary Journal, **57**, 511-512.

Steingrimsson, O, and Alfreosson, G (1982). Campylobacter enteritis in Iceland. Annals of Internal Medicine, **97**, 283-284 [letter].

Stern, N J (1981). Recovery rate of **Campylobacter fetus** ssp. **jejuni** on eviscerated pork, lamb and beef carcasses. Journal of Food Science, **46**, 1291-1293.

Sticht-Groh, V (1982). Campylobacter in healthy slaughter pigs: a possible source of infection for man. Veterinary Record, **110**, 104-106.

Svedhem, A, Kaijser, B, and Sjogren, E (1981). The occurrence of **Campylobacter jejuni** in fresh food and survival under different conditions. Journal of Hygiene, Cambridge, **87**, 421.

Timm, E M, and Wyatt, C J (1981). Incidence of **Campylobacter fetus** subsp. **jejuni** in retail foods. Journal of Food Protection, **44**, 800.

Turnbull, P C B, and Rose, P (1982). **Campylobacter jejuni** and salmonella in raw red meats. Journal of Hygiene, Cambridge, **88**, 29-37.

Weber, V A, Lembke, C, and Kettner, A (1981). Nachweis von **Campylobacter jejuni** in Kotproben von klinisch gesunden Brieftauben [Demonstration of **Campylobacter jejuni** in faeces of clinically normal carrier pigeons]. Berliner und Munchen Tierartzliche Wochenschrift, **94**, 449-451 [English summary].

Wright, E P (1982). The occurrence of **Campylobacter jejuni** in dog faeces from a public park. Journal of Hygiene, Cambridge, **89**, 191-194.

B. SURVIVAL EXPERIMENTS

Blankenship, L C, and Craven, S E (1982). **Campylobacter jejuni** survival in chicken meat as a function of temperature. Applied and Environmental Miccrobiology, **44**, 88-92.

Christopher, F M, Smith, G C, and Vanderzant, C (1982). Effect of temperature and pH on the survival of **Campylobacter fetus**. Journal of

Food Protection, **45**, 253-259 [**C. jejuni** and **C. fetus** subsp. **fetus**]

Doyle, M P, and Roman, D J (1981). Growth and survival of **Campylobacter fetus** subsp. **jejuni** as a function of temperature and pH. Journal of Food Protection, **44**, 596-601.

Doyle, M P, and Roman, D J (1982). Prevalence and survival of **Campylobacter jejuni** in unpasteurized milk. Applied and Environmental Microbiology, **44**, 1154-1158.

Ehlers, J G, Chapparo-Serrano, M, Richter, R L, and Vanderzant, C (1982). Survival of **Campylobacter fetus** subsp. **jejuni** in cheddar and cottage cheese. Journal of Food Protection, **45**, 1018-1021.

Gill, C O, and Harris, L M (1982). Survival and growth of **Campylobacter fetus** subsp. **jejuni** on meat and in cooked foods. Applied and Environmental Microbiology, **44**, 259-263.

Gill, K P W, Bates, P G, and Lander, K P (1981). The effect of pasteurization on the survival of **Campylobacter** species in milk. British Veterinary Journal, **137**, 578-584.

Hanninen, M-L (1981). Survival of **Campylobacter jejuni/coli** in ground refrigerated and in ground frozen beef liver and in frozen broiler carcasses. Acta Veterinaria Scandinavica, **22**, 566-577.

Koidis, P, and Doyle, M P (1983). Survival of **Campylobacter jejuni** in the presence of bisulfite and different atmospheres. European Journal of Clinical Microbiology, **2**, 384-388.

Stern, N J, and Kotula, A W (1982). Survival of **Campylobacter jejuni** inoculated into ground beef. Applied and Environmental Microbiology, **44**, 1150-1153.

Wang, W-L L, Powers, B W, Luechtefeld, N W, and Blaser, M J (1983). Effects of disinfectants on **Campylobacter jejuni**. Applied and Environmental Microbiology, **45**, 1202-1205.

Waterman, S C (1982). The heat-sensitivity of **Campylobacter jejuni** in milk. Journal of Hygiene, Cambridge, **88**, 529-533.

Waterman, S C, and Park, R W A (1982). Survival of **Campylobacter jejuni** and some implications for public health. Journal of Applied Microbiology, **53**, xiii.

Author Index

This index does **not** include any reference to the names of authors of publications listed in the bibliography. It contains the names of all authors who have contributed to or whose work is mentioned in the main text on pp. 1-175.

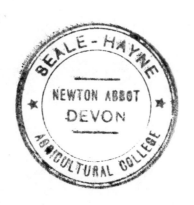